The Successful Physician Negotiator:
How to Get What You Deserve

STEVEN BABITSKY, ESQ.

JAMES J. MANGRAVITI, Jr., ESQ.

S•E•A•K, Inc.
Legal and Medical Information Systems

Falmouth, Massachusetts

The Successful Physician Negotiator:
How to Get What You Deserve
Copyright © 1998 by SEAK, Inc.
ISBN: 0-9652197-7-1

CONTENTS

Preface ix

Acknowledgments xiii

Related Products by SEAK, Inc. xv

About the Authors xvii

Chapter 1 The Physician Negotiator 1

HOW MUCH ARE YOU NEGOTIATING FOR? 1
MORE AT STAKE THAN MONEY 3
WHY PHYSICIANS MAY NOT BE SKILLED NEGOTIATORS 3
WHY PHYSICIANS DON'T NEGOTIATE 7

Chapter 2 Negotiation Basics 11

NEGOTIATION DEFINED 11
COOPERATIVE NEGOTIATIONS: LONG-TERM RELATIONSHIPS .. 12
    Be Assertive 13
    Build Trust 17
    Be on Time 18
    Be Sensitive to Your Opponent's Needs 18
    Emphasize the Benefits of a Long-term Relationship 19
    Build Goodwill 20
    Make a Phone Call 21
    Let People off the Hook 21
COMPETITIVE NEGOTIATION: ONE-SHOT DEALS 22
NEGOTIATION'S "MAGIC" FORMULA 24
THE BEGINNING OF A NEGOTIATION 25
    Ambush Negotiations 27
        Just say no 28
        Ask for it in writing 29

Chapter 3 The Best Place to Negotiate 33

THE HOME FIELD ADVANTAGE 33
HOME FIELD DISADVANTAGE 34
    Interruptions 34
    Unwanted Disclosure of Information 34
    Deflecting Decisions 35

Logistics 36
Preparation and Focus 36
Authors' Recommendation 37

Chapter 4 Controlling and Obtaining Information 39

AUTHORITY 39
    Concessions 42
    Delay 42
    Bargaining against Yourself 43
    Trickle-down Loss 44
    Your Own Authority 44
ASKING QUESTIONS 48
ANSWERING QUESTIONS 57
ACTIVE LISTENING 64
    Equivocal Statements and Verbal Leaks 70
    Body Language 71
    Needs, Interests, and Desires 74

Chapter 5 The Best Time to Negotiate 83

WHEN TO NEGOTIATE 83
PATIENCE AND PAUSING 87
    Patience 87
    Pausing 88
ACCEPTANCE TIME 90
DEADLINES 92
    Deadlines Make Things Happen 92
    Negotiators Respond to and Strive to Meet Deadlines 93
    The Power of Deadlines 94
    Deadlines Play on Your Opponent's Fears 95
    Deadlines Help Reduce Your Opponent's Options 96
    The Pressure of Close Deadlines 97
    The Efficacy of Objective Deadlines 98
    The Extension of Deadlines 99
    The Importance of Accelerated Deadlines 101
CONCLUSION 102

Chapter 6 How to Gain Power in a Negotiation 103

KNOWLEDGE IS POWER 103
ALTERNATIVES 105
INDUSTRY STANDARDS 106
EXPERTISE 107
INVESTMENT 108
LEGITIMACY AND PRECEDENTS 110

COPING WITH UNCERTAINTY 112
PERSISTENCE 113
SOLE SOURCE 115
CONCLUSION 116

Chapter 7 Preparing to Win 117

RECOGNIZE WHEN YOU ARE NEGOTIATING 117
PHYSICIANS ARE TOO BUSY TO PREPARE 118
HOW TO PREPARE 119
 Issues 119
 Goals 120
INFORMATION GATHERING 122
 When 122
 Who 123
 What 124
 Where 125
 Why 126
ANALYSIS 126
 Assumption #1: Your Opponent Will Act as You Would .. 127
 Assumption #2: Your Opponent Will Act Logically 127
 Assumption #3: Your Opponent Will Do What Is in His or
 Her Best Interest 128
PLANNING 129

Chapter 8 Silence Is Golden 133

STRATEGIC WEAPON 133
METHOD OF COMMUNICATION 135
TEMPO 136
CONCLUSION 137

Chapter 9 How to Gain Valuable Concessions 139

ROOM TO NEGOTIATE 139
RECOGNIZING CONCESSIONS 139
VALUE 141
LINKAGE 142
TIMING 144
SIZE AND RATE OF CONCESSIONS 145
INFORMATION AND RATE OF CONCESSIONS 146
THE STORY OF CONCESSIONS 147

Chapter 10 Using and Breaking Deadlock 149

APPEAR WILLING TO WALK AWAY 149
BREAK OR AVOID DEADLOCK 150

Conciliatory Language.. 150
Flexibility 151
Adequate Room to Negotiate 152
Deadlines and Ultimatums 153
Eliminating the Possibility of Deadlock 154
Change 156
CONCLUSION... 160

Chapter 11 Using Controlled Emotions to Your Advantage 161

PLAYING IT COOL 161
Diffusing the Opponent 162
CONTROLLING YOUR ANGER... 163
Personalize the Negotiation.. 164
TAPPING INTO FEAR OR ANXIETY..................................... 165
CONCLUSION... 168

Chapter 12 Telephone Negotiations................................... 169

CONCENTRATE AND FOCUS.. 169
PREPARE... 170
INITIATE THE CALL... 171
LISTEN FOR AUDITORY FEEDBACK..................................... 173
TAKE NOTES AND SEND CONFIRMATION LETTERS.............. 174
CONCLUSION... 175

Chapter 13 Defeating Your Opponent's Tactics.................. 177

TACTIC 1: LET'S SPLIT THE DIFFERENCE 177
TACTIC 2: TAKE IT OR LEAVE IT 179
TACTIC 3: THE ESTIMATE: BALLPARK PRICE....................... 183
TACTIC 4: LACK OF CANDOR 186
TACTIC 5: OUTRAGEOUS OPENING OFFER OR DEMAND........ 189
TACTIC 6: BELLY UP 190
TACTIC 7: ANCHORING... 191
TACTIC 8: YOU HAVE GOT TO DO BETTER THAN THAT 193
TACTIC 9: PLEADING POVERTY... 194
TACTIC 10: LIMITED AUTHORITY....................................... 196
ADDITIONAL TACTICS 197

Chapter 14 Team Negotiating.. 201

SIZE AND COMPOSITION OF THE TEAM 201
CONTROLLING THE INFORMATION FLOW 202
GOAL SETTING.. 204
SIGNALING.. 205
TAKING NOTES 207

CAUCUSING... 208
RESOLVING TEAM DISAGREEMENTS..................................... 210
TEAM NEGOTIATION TACTICS... 211
   Divide and Conquer.. 211
   Weak Link.. 212
AGENDAS.. 214
FLEXIBILITY.. 215

Chapter 15 Negotiating for the Retention of an Attorney ... 217

LAW OFFICE ECONOMICS.. 217
LEGAL FEE ARRANGEMENTS.. 220
   Contingency Fee.. 221
   Fixed Fee.. 224
   Hourly Fee... 225
      1. Ask for a reduced hourly rate............................225
      2. Ask for a reduced rate for associates' time and travel.......226
      3. Get an estimate of total cost...........................226
      4. Request billing by the tenth of the hour...........................226
      5. Set a maximum fee not to be exceeded.........................227
      6. Ask for reduced charges for standard forms and agreements
     227
      7. Request weekly or monthly itemized billing....................227
      8. Request efficient handling of the case ("Ask or ye may not
      receive")...228
      9. Request reduced billing for attorney conferences and for file
      reviews...228
      10. Strive to resolve the case by settlement or alternative
      dispute resolution before incurring large legal bills.............228
EXPENSES... 229
WHEN TO HIRE AN ATTORNEY.. 230
HOW TO BE A GOOD CLIENT AND MAKE IT PAY OFF 231
SELECTION OF COUNSEL.. 233

**Chapter 16 Negotiating Employment, Managed Care, and
Other Formal Written Contracts.................................... 235**

CONTRACT LAW.. 235
   State Specific... 235
   Interpretation... 236
   Damages.. 236
IMPORTANT CONTRACTUAL CLAUSES 237
   Choice of Forum Clause....................................... 237
   Choice of Law Clause... 238
   Arbitration Clause... 239
   Indemnity Clauses.. 241
   Limitation of Liability Clause............................... 242

Covenants Not to Compete 242
Liquidated Damages Clauses 244
Force Majeure 245
Severability 245
Notice 246
Assignment 247
Termination 247
NON-FORM CONTRACTS 247
NEGOTIATING STANDARD FORM CONTRACTS........................ 252

Chapter 17 Closing the Deal **257**

ASSUMPTIVE CLOSE 257
LINKAGE.. 258
CLEAR CHOICE.. 259
POWER OF INVESTMENT 260
HAVING A DEAL... 261
Outstanding Issues.. 262
Written Memoranda and Contracts.............................. 263
Living up to the Agreement... 264
FACE SAVING... 265
AN ALTERNATIVE APPROACH.. 266

Resources.. **269**

Index.. **279**

Preface

The authors have over 30 years combined experience in negotiating with, against, and on behalf of physicians. We have reached some striking conclusions. The first two are:

> 1. the majority of physicians are poor negotiators, and
> 2. physicians who are good negotiators are more financially successful and secure than their counterparts.

Another finding we made is that, for reasons we will discuss shortly, physicians frequently do not even attempt to negotiate for themselves. For example, let's say that you are asked by your church or civic organization to purchase $5,000 worth of food for a function. Would you go to your local supermarket and just load up a cart and pay for the food? Probably not. You would most likely feel an obligation to look for the best deal or at least negotiate a better price. Why would you do that? Your reasons may include the following.

> 1. You know your church or civic organization does not have any extra money to waste.
> 2. You feel that you have a special obligation to do the best you can for your organization.
> 3. You know you can get a better price if you try.
> 4. When you get a better price it will make you feel good about yourself and what you have accomplished for your organization.
> 5. You are not embarrassed or uncomfortable with negotiating on behalf of a charity.

6. You will devote the time needed to get a good deal because it is for charitable purposes.

When physicians negotiate in their practices or in personal purchases, they are in fact negotiating for themselves and their families. Should these physicians be any less aggressive or diligent in their negotiating? The authors would suggest that the answer is clearly and emphatically no.

As a preliminary matter, physicians need to accept the following three important premises about negotiating.

1. They and their families have no extra money to waste.
2. They are under a special obligation to their families to do the best they can for them.
3. They very often can get better prices and deals when they try.

Seeking the best price or deal should not make physicians uncomfortable or embarrassed. It should, on the contrary, give them pride and satisfaction in knowing that they have done the best they could for themselves and their families. This is the kind of attitude that physicians need to be successful negotiators.

Many physicians do not negotiate effectively due to a lack of understanding of the process and/or because they are uncomfortable, embarrassed, and lack the skill set or mindset to do so. This point was driven home in a graphic fashion when the authors witnessed a physician purchase a $250,000 piece of real estate. The negotiation between the doctor and the realtor was so short that it should be in the Guinness *Book of World Records*. Here is a verbatim transcript of the entire negotiation after the doctor was told of the $250,000 price:

Doctor:	Can I negotiate?
Realtor:	No.

This four-word "negotiation" concluded with the purchase of the $250,000 piece of property at the full asking price.[*]

Physicians are notoriously poor negotiators despite being highly intelligent and highly educated. One important reason for this lack of negotiating skill is the lack of training physicians receive in this critical area. This text was written to bridge the gap between what physicians presently know about negotiating and what they need to know to be successful and to get what they deserve. With the use of this text, the physician will understand the negotiation process, set realistic goals, and negotiate from a position of power and strength. Do you as a physician owe any less to yourself and your family?

Steven Babitsky, Esq.
James J. Mangraviti, Jr., Esq.

---

[*] The story does have a happy ending—the value of the property has (fortunately) doubled since the purchase.

Acknowledgments

The authors wish to acknowledge their partner, Christopher R. Brigham, MD, without whom this book would not have been possible. The authors would also like to acknowledge Dee Netzel for her fine work in copy editing and typesetting this work in the face of an extremely tight time deadline.

Related Products by SEAK, Inc.

AUDIOTAPE PROGRAMS
Achieving Success with Workers' Compensation

Achieving Success as a Medical Witness

TEXTS
The Independent Medical Examination Report:
A Step-by-Step Guide with Models

How to Excel During Cross-Examination:
Techniques for Experts that Work

The Comprehensive IME System: Essential Resources
for an Efficient and Successful IME Practice

For more information call SEAK at 508/457-1111.
Inquiries may also be addressed to SEAK, Inc. at
P.O. Box 729, Falmouth, MA 02541. Fax 508/540-
8304; e-mail address: seakinc@aol.com; Internet
address: http://www.seak.com

About the Authors

Steven Babitsky, Esq., is the president of SEAK, Inc. He was a personal injury trial attorney for 20 years and has over 25 years experience as a professional negotiator. Attorney Babitsky is the editor of *The Expert Witness Journal* and the seminar leader for the National Expert Witness and Litigation Seminar. Attorney Babitsky is the co-author of the text *How to Excel During Cross-Examination: Techniques for Experts that Work.* He has produced 13 medical/legal training videos over the past two years. Attorney Babitsky is the co-developer and trainer for the "Negotiation Skills for Physicians" seminar.

James J. Mangraviti, Jr., Esq., is a former trial lawyer with experience in defense and plaintiff personal injury law and insurance law. He currently serves as vice-president and general counsel of SEAK, Inc. Mr. Mangraviti received his B.A. degree in mathematics *summa cum laude* from Boston College and his JD degree *cum laude* from Boston College Law School. His publications include the texts *The Independent Medical Examination Report: A Step-by-Step Guide with Models* and *How to Excel During Cross-Examination: Techniques for Experts that Work.* Mr. Mangraviti has lectured extensively to physicians across the United States.

Chapter 1 The Physician Negotiator

How Much Are You Negotiating For?

As a physician, you can expect to negotiate for *millions* of dollars over the course of your career. Consider Box 1.1, below.

Box 1.1

Typical Physician Negotiations over 20 Years	
Salary	$4,000,000
Salaries of Staff	$1,500,000
Purchase of Homes	$750,000
Sale of Home	$350,000
Automobile Purchases	$100,000
Automobile Sales	$50,000
Legal Fees	$100,000
Accounting Fees	$100,000
Equipment Purchases	$200,000
Consumer Goods	$300,000
Total: $7,450,000	

As you can see in this very conservative example, an average physician negotiates for tremendously large amounts of money over just 20 years of his or her career. Taking the example in Box 1.1, consider what would happen if the physician could save just 5% of this total. Five percent of $7,450,000 amounts to over $370,000. If the physician could save

10%, the savings would be approximately $750,000 (three-quarters of a million dollars)!

To appreciate how much you as a physician have at stake in learning to negotiate, consider approximately how much you will be negotiating for over the next 20 years. You can use Box 1.2 as a worksheet to arrive at a rough approximation.

Box 1.2

Negotiations over the Next 20 Years	
Salary	$_____
Salaries of Staff	$_____
Purchase of Homes	$_____
Sale of Home	$_____
Automobile Purchases	$_____
Automobile Sales	$_____
Legal Fees	$_____
Accounting Fees	$_____
Equipment Purchases	$_____
Consumer Goods	$_____
Other	$_____
Other	$_____
Total: $_____	

The purpose of this book is to empower physicians to save an average of 5% to 10% when negotiating. Multiply the total from Box 1.2 by .05 and .10 to determine how much you can save over the next 20 years through more skilled and effective negotiating. Saving 5%, 10%, or more requires superior negotiating skills. This book has been designed to help physicians develop such skills.

<u>More at Stake than Money</u>

There are other important reasons why you should develop superior negotiating skills. First, superior negotiating skills will allow you to feel more comfortable during negotiations. Second, the assertiveness that is required of a savvy negotiator will help you in other aspects of your professional and personal life. Finally, once you have developed superior negotiating skills, you will be able to increase the level of satisfaction you have with the purchases and agreements you make.

<u>Why Physicians May Not Be Skilled Negotiators</u>

In general, physicians have the reputation of being poor negotiators and business people. There are many reasons for this. First and foremost is a lack of training in negotiation skills. Physicians are some of the most highly educated and trained professionals. Typically, not one minute of this training and education involves negotiation skills. Negotiation skills courses are offered by SEAK, Inc. and many other adult education organizations. A wise physician will further his or her skills and take one.

Another reason that physicians are poor negotiators is that they are trained from internship on to follow the instructions of their teachers, mentors, and superiors. They are also trained to be responsive to patients' needs and to help them get better. The mindset that often develops after many years of intensive training is that confrontations with superiors, colleagues, and patients should be avoided. Physicians are told that if they do not fall into line, they risk getting labeled as difficult, thus jeopardizing their careers.

Example 1.1
Employer: The job pays $110,000 per year, okay?
Doctor: Ahh..., well, the going rate for my specialty in this part of the country is $130,000.
Employer: Look, we need team players here. We're all on the same team, right? You want to be a team player, don't you, just like Doctors Smith and Jones?
Doctor: Of course.
Employer: Okay then, the players on this team are paid $110,000, a very handsome salary, and they don't complain, they mind their own business, and they don't worry about what other people are doing.
Doctor: (embarrassed) Okay.

Lesson: To become successful negotiators, physicians must accept the fact that confrontation with the other party (i.e., the opponent in a negotiation) is sometimes necessary. The physician's unwillingness to be assertive in this case may have cost him $20,000 per year, or $100,000 over five years.

As attorneys, the authors accept the premise that confrontation is *not* something inherently evil or to be ashamed of. If we did not, we would not meet our ethical obligation to represent zealously the interests of our clients. As a physician, you also need to accept the fact that there is nothing wrong with standing up for yourself and your family and trying to obtain a fair deal. Doctors who learn to be assertive earn the respect of their peers and opponents and are generally more successful than doctors who are not assertive. Take as an example how a physician might have better handled the situation in Example 1.1.

Example 1.2
Employer: The job pays $110,000 per year, okay?
Doctor: No, I'm sorry that's unacceptable. The going rate for my specialty in this part of the country is $130,000.
Employer: Look, we need team players here. We're all on the same team, right? You want to be a team player, don't you, just like Doctors Smith and Jones?
Doctor: I am a team player and very much look forward to being part of your team. However, I need to be paid what I'm worth, and what I'm worth is $130,000. You don't want an unhappy team member, do you?
Employer: Okay then, $130,000. We believe very strongly in paying our team members what they think they're worth.
Doctor: (enthusiastic) Okay. When do I start?

Lesson: The physician was able to get the salary she was seeking by being assertive and *asking* for it. Also note that the physician was not afraid to say no to the employer's low-ball offer of $110,000. The ability to say no is another extremely important skill that the savvy negotiator needs to master. (See pages 28-29 on saying no.)

    Another reason that physicians are poor negotiators is their mindset, which many times includes the need to be liked. Some physicians do not like to negotiate because they don't want to be a "bad guy." Worse, they consciously or subconsciously give away everything in an effort to make sure that the person they are negotiating with likes them. A desire to be liked is natural. A *need* to be liked is understandable, but it can be extremely detrimental when negotiating. An opponent will quickly detect this weakness and use it against the physician. To be a successful physician negotiator, your primary focus should be on the deal under negotiation. If the goal is, instead, being liked by the opponent, the physician is heading for serious trouble.

Take as an example a person who negotiates professionally, say an attorney. Would you want an attorney who was representing you to be worried about whether the opponent would like him or her at the conclusion of the negotiation? The answer is clearly NO! You would want the attorney to use his or her negotiating skills, experience, and training to get you the best agreement or deal possible. Attorneys are successful during negotiating because they temporarily repress their human desire to be liked. Physicians need to do the same if they want to be successful negotiators. Consider the following example.

Example 1.3
Salesman: (friendly and enthusiastically) Hi, doctor. How's the family?
Doctor: Fine, thanks.
Salesman: What did you think of that game last night?
Doctor: That was something else, wasn't it?
Salesman: Yeah, it was. So are you ready to move on that Audi?
Doctor: Love to, but would it be possible to knock another two grand off the price?
Salesman: (taken aback and quiet) I thought we'd settled all that. I gave you a price of $32,000 and you didn't have a problem with it.
Doctor: (unsure) Yeah, but my wife thought it was a bit high.

Salesman: (sadly) If I don't close this sale at the price we had previously talked about, my sales manager is going to be furious. I already told him we had a deal, which is what I thought. My wife will kill me if I lose this job. She's expecting, you know.

Doctor: Okay, let's do it at $32,000.

Salesman: (friendly again) Doctor Jones, you're the best.

Lesson: Had Dr. Jones stood firm and not been concerned with his opponent's desires and with his own need to be liked, he would have been much more likely to purchase the car for the price he wanted.

Why Physicians Don't Negotiate

There are many reasons physicians use to justify their failure to negotiate. The five most common excuses are that:

1. they do not have the time,
2. they are embarrassed,
3. they do not feel comfortable negotiating,
4. they do not like conflict or disagreement, and
5. they feel that asserting themselves during negotiations is not professional.

To be a successful physician negotiator you need to move beyond these excuses. Consider Box 1.3.

Box 1.3

Physician Excuses Not to Negotiate

1. *I don't have enough time.* To be a successful physician negotiator you need to devote the time needed to negotiating. There is simply too much at stake—millions of dollars (see pages 1-2), to not devote an appropriate amount of time to negotiating. If your schedule is tight, you need to make the time to negotiate. (See pages 118-119 on making time to negotiate.)

2. *It's embarrassing.* As a physician you have trained intensively for years, paid for a very expensive education, and worked long hours under stressful conditions. You should not be embarrassed to ask for what you deserve.

3. *I don't feel comfortable.* This is a natural reaction. The way you develop a level of comfort is to learn about the negotiation process, to understand the tactics and defenses, and to actually negotiate a few times. It's just like riding a bike. The toughest part is doing it the first few times, then you are comfortable and never forget how to do it.

4. *I don't like conflict or disagreement.* This is a feeling shared by many physicians. Unfortunately, in order to be a successful physician negotiator, you must suppress this feeling during negotiations. Courteous and professional disagreement is a necessary part of most, if not all, negotiations.

5. *It's not professional.* This is simply not true. There is nothing unprofessional about standing up for yourself and your family and asserting yourself during negotiations.

There is no need for physicians to continue to fall into the trap of viewing negotiating as unprofessional. Consider the following example.

Example 1.4
Opponent: (to doctor) You are being very demanding. I have dealt with dozens of other doctors and none of them has ever asked for changes in this PPO agreement.
Doctor: I'm not concerned with other doctors. What I am concerned with is maintaining the highest quality level of care for my patients and making sure that I am fairly compensated for my services.

Lesson: Asserting your right to be treated fairly is simply not unprofessional!

Chapter 2 Negotiation Basics

Negotiation Defined

The great commentator Edwin R. Murrow once said, "the term *negotiation* implies compromise; painful concessions on the part of both parties." A sterile definition of *negotiation* is to confer and to discuss to reach an agreement. The experts describe negotiation as a more fluid, complex process that involves our most basic needs and desires:

> Negotiation is the field of knowledge and endeavors that focuses on gaining the favor of people from whom we want things. We want all sorts of things: prestige, freedom, money, justice, love, status, security, and recognition. What is negotiation? It is the use of information and power to affect behavior within a web of tension.... A negotiation is more than an exchange of material objects. It is a way of acting and behaving that can develop understanding, belief, acceptance, respect, and trust. It is the manner of your approach, the tone of your voice, the attitude you convey, the methods you use, and the concern you exhibit for the other side's feelings and needs.[1]

Thus, negotiation is a process that typically involves:

- an exchange of material objects,
- the use of power and information to affect behavior,

---

[1] Herb Cohen, *You Can Negotiate Anything: How to Get What You Want* (Secaucus, NJ: Carol Publishing Group, 1996) 15, 154.

- communication to obtain approval, agreement, or action of another party, and
- gaining the favor of people from whom you want things.

Negotiation is a fascinating and challenging art and skill. It requires the ability to recognize the complexities of human nature and its desires and the ability to satisfy both your needs and the needs of the person you are negotiating with. Physicians should use their insight into, and their professional training concerning, human behavior to achieve more favorable agreements. Physicians should not dread negotiation; they should look at it as an intellectual challenge.

Cooperative Negotiations: Long-term Relationships

Most negotiation experts agree that the two major types of negotiations are cooperative negotiations and competitive negotiations. This section will explain how physicians can differentiate between these two types of negotiation and why it is crucial to be able to do so.

The cooperative negotiation is characterized by an exchange of information in which there is give and take. A participant in a cooperative negotiation asks questions to find out what is important to the person he or she is negotiating with. The search is for a "win-win" solution or agreement in which both parties gain and are satisfied with the outcome. Particular emphasis is placed on creating new business opportunities, synergy, and the distinct possibility of future agreements and business if things go well.

This type of negotiation is of particular importance to physicians because they frequently negotiate for the long term (i.e., with colleagues, health-care providers, insurers, and other professionals with whom they will most likely continue to do business with). Your ability to distinguish cooperative from competitive negotiation and to change a potentially competitive negotiation into a cooperative one are skills of the successful physician negotiator.

When negotiating, we are not looking for a single short-term deal in which we make the most profit and pay as little as possible. We emphasize that we are looking for a way to pay the opponent as much as possible and still make a good profit for ourselves. Using this philosophy, we can gain important concessions from the opponent and establish a long-term relationship in which both parties are satisfied and where multiple future projects are possible. What could be a competitive negotiation is turned into a cooperative win-win agreement by stressing the desire for a long-term relationship and making sure that the opponent gets a good deal.

The cooperative problem-solving approach to negotiations is characterized by a genuine search for the best deal for both parties. This approach involves being forthright with the disclosure of information, the use of reasonable opening demands or requests, and honest, courteous, sincere dialogue designed to achieve a win-win solution. When this approach is used correctly, the parties do not fight about how to divide the pie, but look for and find mutually agreeable ways to make a bigger pie to divide.

BE ASSERTIVE

As a physician negotiator you face challenges that are not often encountered by other professionals. Your long years of medical training have stressed collaboration, cooperation, and team building. Individualism has been discouraged. The training you received in medical school, your internship, and your residency may have left you deferential to authority, accepting of the standard way physicians do things, unquestioning, trusting, passive, and unwilling or unable to be assertive on your own behalf. If you possess one or more of these traits you will have to overcome them to become a more effective physician negotiator. You must believe and act on the knowledge that just because someone in authority says something, this does not mean that the terms must be accepted as presented.

Example 2.1
Doctor: How often will I be on call?
Administrator: Three weekends a month.
Doctor: Why so many?
Administrator: That is the way we have been doing it for 35 years.
Doctor: I appreciate your long-standing policy, but unfortunately that does not work for me. My husband and I just had our first child and I cannot give up three weekends per month....

Lesson: For the physician to have any hope of getting better terms than being on call three weekends per month, she could not let the negotiation end on the administrator's statement that that's the way the hospital's done things for 35 years. The doctor's ability to question the status quo was a prerequisite to gaining favorable terms.

Remember that the status quo is just a starting point and should not necessarily be your final destination. One quick way for you to become more assertive is to think not of what the additional money or time will mean for you, but of what it will mean for your children, spouse, extended family, etc. In a very real sense you are negotiating for them as well. The extra money or time you can obtain will go for education, lessons, family time, vacations, and a safe environment.

You may feel very uncomfortable when your negotiation involves a long-term relationship. This is natural. You will often negotiate with colleagues and you do not want to make an enemy or alienate a person with whom you will have to deal with in the future. You want to be a team player and not a troublemaker. Many physicians fear that being too assertive is unprofessional. They are wrong. Your opponents know about your fears regarding confrontation and assertiveness and will use them against you.

Example 2.2
Hospital administrator: Doctor, as I understand it, all the other physicians on staff are on call one night a week but you feel this schedule should not apply to you.

Lesson: To be a superior physician negotiator, the doctor in this example must not be afraid to say, "Yes. I can't follow the schedule kept by the other doctors." If the doctor doesn't ask, he will never receive.

Example 2.3
Employer: (to prospective new physician employee) We all started with these terms. The key is to get you started and on the team. The beginning of the relationship is not the time to rock the boat.... So, please sign this seven-year employment contract.

Lesson: This is a snow job. The doctor needs to assert herself if she is going to get what she deserves. One response the doctor could use could be, "I look forward to formally joining the team, but I can't commit to seven years of employment with your group, or any other group, unless we settle these issues up front. Now, as we discussed, my requirements in terms of vacation time are as follows...."

The key to success in negotiating long-term relationships is to be assertive enough to suggest a better deal for both parties and to invent options for mutual gain. In short, you need to look for a win-win solution.[2] A physician who has become a skilled negotiator will recognize that these win-win opportunities are available but that they need to be searched for and advocated. Once you look for the creative solutions that satisfy the needs of all the parties, you are no longer negotiating "against" an opponent. You are now both working together to find a win-win solution. This is a concept that may be counterintuitive. You can be aggressive and assertive but still build amicable long-term relationships. You need to recognize that many times the potential long-term relationship is as important as the negotiation itself and that you will most likely gain, not lose, respect by being assertive.

When dealing with long-term relationships you need to be concerned with how satisfied your opponent

---

[2] "Far too many of us, when we are involved in a conflict, think mainly—or only—of the 'win,' when our best interests would be served if we thought instead of the relationship with the person with whom we are experiencing the conflict." Fred E. Jandt, *Win-Win Negotiating: Turning Conflict into Agreement* (New York: John Wiley & Sons, 1985) 135.

is with the result of the negotiation. There are two reasons for this. First, you want your opponent to be amenable to future agreements and projects. Second, you want her to enthusiastically live up to the agreement in a timely fashion. (See pages 264-265 on living up to the agreement.)

Win-win negotiation is not a game with winners and losers. It is the first step in building a long-term relationship based on trust, respect, integrity, and agreements that work well for both sides. As a successful physician negotiator you want to expand your business relationships, not waste your time continually searching for new ones.[3] Various ways to expand your existing business relationships are discussed in the next several subsections.

BUILD TRUST

Building trust is very important when dealing with long-term relationships. Trust is built over time. If you develop the reputation as a "straight shooter"—a person of your word—this will make your negotiations easier and less stressful. If you can build a mutually trusting relationship, the question will be changed from if you can reach an agreement to how it will be accomplished.

---

[3] "Expanding on an existing business relationship is almost always easier than starting a new one. By creating the right impression you make people want to deal with you over and over again. Achieving that often comes down to knowing how hard to push." Mark H. McCormack, *What They Don't Teach You at Harvard Business School: Notes from A Street Smart Executive* (New York: Bantam Books, 1984) 41.

Example 2.4
Publisher: Can you have the book done by June 1, 1999?
Doctor: No, but realistically I will have it on your desk on July 28, 1999.

Lesson: By being honest, direct, and not promising more than she can deliver, the doctor has built trust with the publisher.

BE ON TIME

It is rare to see high quality work done in a timely fashion. Any reputation you build for this type of performance will be a great asset during the ongoing negotiations of a long-term relationship.

Example 2.5
Doctor: You don't question the fact that my work will be high quality and delivered on time, do you?
Opponent: Not for a minute!

Lesson: The doctor, by pointing out that both parties agree that her work will be timely and of high quality, has made it much harder for the opponent to argue that the work is not as valuable as the doctor says it is.

BE SENSITIVE TO YOUR OPPONENT'S NEEDS

You should be sensitive to the needs, desires, and concerns of the person you are negotiating with. If you can communicate this sensitivity to your opponents, they will be more likely to trust you. Also, understanding your opponent is critical when you need to obtain a deal that is a "win" for both sides.

Example 2.6
Doctor: (to opponent) What would work best for you? *(or)* Let's see how we can get you what you need.

Lesson: This query should be helpful in building trust and making a win-win deal more possible.

EMPHASIZE THE BENEFITS OF A LONG-TERM RELATIONSHIP

You should almost always stress the fact that a relationship will be long term. This will accomplish at least two things. First, you will remind your opponent that he or she has more at stake than this one deal. Second, you can communicate that it is in *your opponent's* best interest to treat you fairly and make sure you are happy.

Example 2.7
Doctor: (to colleague) Doctor, as you know, it is my hope, if we can work things out satisfactorily, that this is the first of many projects we will be working on together.
Colleague: Absolutely. Once we get this project done....

Lesson: By stressing that she is seeking a long-term relationship, the doctor has communicated that there is more at stake here than the one project. She has also communicated that future projects are dependent upon the deal obtained in this project.

BUILD GOODWILL

In a potential long-term relationship, people want to associate themselves with people they trust and like. If you can establish goodwill, your negotiations will be less stressful and more profitable. A great way to build goodwill is to do a favor for your opponent.

Example 2.8
Doctor (employer): I see here that you're a golfer.
New physician employee: Yes, it's my third passion after medicine and my family.
Doctor: Have you played the Mountain View Club?
New physician employee: No, that's private. I've been dying to get in there.
Doctor: I'm on the executive committee of that club. Been a member for 28 years. I can sponsor you for membership. I'll give them a call right now....

Lesson: When it comes time to renegotiate the physician's employment contract or when it becomes time to buy into the practice, the new employee will remember the doctor's unsolicited act regarding the country club. The negotiations will be easier.

Example 2.9
The authors put on seminars all across the United States. At one seminar a medical book publisher was a paid exhibitor. He was a one-man operation and was there by himself. After the completion of a three-day program we were all exhausted. As we walked out of the door, we spotted this exhibitor struggling to pack all of his books into a truck. We asked if he needed assistance and spent 20 minutes helping him. He thanked us again and again and has become a friend to

this day. Seven years later we still do business together. With this small favor we showed him (as opposed to telling him) that we were easy to deal with, friendly, and cooperative. When given an opportunity, demonstrating is far more effective than telling someone the same thing.

MAKE A PHONE CALL

Frequently, a simple phone call to share some information is all it takes to help build a long-term relationship.

Example 2.10

You want to merge with another group. You have had informal discussions about this merger with the doctor who heads the other group. You know that the group wants to change its office location. The real estate market is very tight. You become aware of some ideal space that is available and call up the other group's head to let her know. She really appreciated it. The cost was minimal but the goodwill benefits could be enormous if and when merger negotiations resume.

LET PEOPLE OFF THE HOOK

If you notice that the person you are negotiating with makes an error or if circumstances beyond the person's control have changed, point it out promptly. This is especially true in the short term if it would work to your advantage to say nothing. You should be careful about mentioning these favors later because neither side is likely to forget them and it may embarrass the other side.

Example 2.11
When negotiating a contract for a series of medical
videos, we noted that the physician we were negotiating
with made a mathematical error, which would have
worked to our advantage. We pulled him aside and
gently pointed out his error. This saved him from a
major problem with his employer and, as you might
expect, he really appreciated it. Trust was built and we
have been dealing with that physician ever since.

Competitive Negotiation: One-Shot Deals

The competitive negotiation is characterized by the
desire to win. It usually does not involve a long-term
relationship. In a competitive negotiation, your
opponent will disclose as little information as possible,
show little concern for the other party, attempt to
manipulate the situation, and use every negotiation
tactic possible to achieve the best result for him- or
herself. An example of a competitive negotiation is a
onetime purchase, such as an automobile.

In sharp contrast to cooperative negotiations,
people involved in competitive negotiation are more apt
to misstate the truth and be skeptical about any
assertions you make. In competitive negotiations, the
opening demands may be unrealistic and every action
and statement of the parties after that are designed to
achieve one thing only—to win. The use of threats,
posturing, and hardball tactics are all frequently part of
competitive negotiation.

Successful physician negotiators must be able to
quickly recognize whether they are involved in a
competitive or a cooperative negotiation. Savvy
physician negotiators attempt to move from a
competitive to a cooperative negotiation by asking the
simple question, "How do we come up with a better

deal for both of us?" Once both parties begin this search, they have moved toward a cooperative negotiation. This ability to change negotiations from competitive to cooperative will be especially helpful in building long-term relationships. Consider Example 2.12 in which the doctor converts a competitive negotiation into a cooperative negotiation through forthrightness and the promise of future business.

Example 2.12

Doctor: I'm interested in that new Toyota.

Salesman: Step into my office and let's do a work up.

Doctor: Okay, but before you do the work up I want you to know a few things. I'm here to buy a Toyota. My family drives Toyotas. I have a wife and two teenage children that I will also be buying Toyotas for over the next couple of years. I have done my homework and I know exactly what you pay the manufacturer for this model. I can pay you 5% over invoice, which is a fair margin for you. I'm not here to get something for nothing; you deserve a fair profit. However, I don't want to haggle or play games here. If you treat me correctly and respectfully you'll have us for customers for years to come. By my calculations 5% over invoice is $22,456.

Salesman: I appreciate your candor and forthrightness and look forward to serving your family for years to come. You've got yourself a deal.

Doctor: I look forward to working with you as well. When can I take delivery?

Lesson: Not only was the doctor able to secure himself a fair deal, but he was also able to defuse a potentially hostile negotiation and make his future car buying negotiations relatively stress free.

Negotiation's "Magic" Formula

What is the "formula" for becoming a successful physician negotiator? Unfortunately, it is not as simple as deciphering the fictitious formula in Box 2.1 and applying it to your situation.

Box 2.1

Negotiation Formula
$I + P + K = SN$

In fact, negotiation is an extremely complex art. There is no quick, simple, and easy formula for becoming a successful physician negotiator. To be a superior physician negotiator you need to understand all of the negotiation principles contained in Box 2.2. You will also need to apply the principles to your everyday negotiations.

Box 2.2

Negotiation Principles	
Agendas	Introduction
Aspiration levels	Listening skills
Authority	Long-term relationships
Body language	Mutual gain
Characteristics/negotiator	Negotiation location
Clarity of language	Objectives
Closings	Opponent's desires
Communication	Opponent's motives
Competitive negotiations	Power
Concessions	Preparation
Control	Principled negotiations
Cooperative negotiations	Questions
Correspondence	Quickie negotiations

Counteroffers	Relationships
Deadlines	Setting targets
Deadlock	Silence
Defenses	Tactics
Emotions	Take it or leave it
Exercises	Telephone negotiations
Goals	Threats
Goodwill	Time as a weapon
Group negotiating	Ultimatums
Habits	What makes people act
Information	Win-win
Interests	

The Beginning of a Negotiation

The most fundamental skill that you will need to develop is to recognize when a negotiation has begun. *Any* communication with another person who you may deal with in the future should be considered part of a negotiation. This is especially true when information is sought or given. Thus, you need to be very careful about disclosing information that could be used against you by a person who may want to do business with you. Consider Example 2.13.

Example 2.13
Setting: A cocktail party

Background: The physician is employed by Group X, hates it, and is desperate to get out. Group Y needs a new physician and is willing to pay up to $175,000/year. The national average salary for the physician's specialty is $150,000.

Head of Group Y: So, how do you like things over at Group X?

Doctor: It's terrible. I'm looking to move.

Head of Group Y: Sorry to hear that. Are they paying you competitively?

Doctor: Not even, I'm about 10% under the national average.

Head of Group Y: Well, I hope everything works out for you.

Epilogue: One week later, the head of Group Y calls the doctor and "starts" negotiations to bring him into the group. The doctor agrees to switch for $150,000/year. The negotiation began at the party. The doctor's revelation of information hurt him later.

Lesson: The negotiation did *not* begin when the head of the group called the physician one week after the party. It began with the disclosure of information by the doctor to the head of the group at the party. In one brief conversation the doctor disclosed the crucial information of what he was paid and that he hated his present job. His opponent disclosed next to nothing. The result was devastating in that the physician accepted a job for $25,000/year less than what he could have received from the new employer. Note that once the damaging information was disclosed by the doctor, there was very little that could be done to repair the damage. If the doctor in this example had been savvy enough to recognize that a negotiation was possibly beginning, he could have withheld the damaging information.

Example 2.14
Setting: A cocktail party

Background: The physician is employed by Group X, hates it, and is desperate to get out. Group Y needs a new physician and is willing to pay up to $175,000/year. The national average salary for the physician's specialty is $150,000.

Head of Group Y: So, how do you like things over at Group X?
Doctor: Why do you ask?
Head of Group Y: We're looking for new staffing.
Doctor: Really. What's the pay?
Head of Group Y: Very competitive.
Doctor: Give me a call next week and we can talk more about it.

Epilogue: One week later, the head of Group Y calls the doctor and starts negotiations to bring him into the group. The doctor agrees to switch for $175,000/year.

Lesson: The doctor's negotiating skills, his ability to control the disclosure of damaging information, and his ability to obtain important information from his opponent will make him an extra $125,000 over five years.

AMBUSH NEGOTIATIONS

Many physicians do not properly identify a telephone call or a casual remark as the beginning of the negotiation process. This is what we call the *ambush negotiation.* You need to understand that once someone has asked you, "Will you be able to...," you are in the midst of a rapidly developing negotiation. Be

very careful about agreeing to requests without first
determining:

1. the effort that will be involved,
2. whether the work will have to be done at
home and at night,
3. if you will have to give up or postpone more
important or lucrative work to accomplish the
tasks involved,
4. if you really have the time to do this project,
5. if you will have to give up family time or
much-needed recreation or vacation time to
complete the task, and perhaps most
importantly,
6. whether or not you really want to do this
project.

Example 2.15
Publisher: Doctor, will you be able to write a brief
chapter on (fill in the physician's area of specialty or
expertise) for the text we are working on?
Doctor: Sure, no problem. Happy to do it!

Lesson: This is an ambush negotiation in which a
physician has been taken by surprise. The physician
has committed himself to many hours of hard work
without any consideration of the time and effort
involved, adequate compensation, deadlines, and work
or family time that will have to be sacrificed to meet
this new commitment.

Just say no
Your ability to say no can save you hundreds of hours a
year. However, many physicians have great difficulty
in just saying no. The ability to just say no or to deflect

and postpone a decision until you are provided with the details and do a little thinking is crucial if you want to be a superior physician negotiator.

Example 2.16
Publisher: Doctor, will you be able to write a brief chapter for the text we are working on?
Doctor: I'm sorry, I can't.

Lesson: The ability to say no is imperative. Having this ability will save you time, aggravation, and money.

Ask for it in writing
One technique you can use to avoid being ambushed is to ask for the proposal in writing. This type of reply will accomplish several things. First, it will reduce the time spent on many preliminary requests (i.e., the feeling-out type of requests that just waste physicians' time). Second, it will give a physician time to think about whether he really wants to do the project. Finally, it will provide the physician with the information he needs to decide if the project is financially and professionally in his best interest.

Example 2.17
Publisher: Will you be able to write a brief chapter for the text we are working on?
Doctor: It sounds interesting. Please send me a note with the details—what you are looking for in terms of length, content, original research, time deadlines, format, my compensation, and the compensation of the other authors and editors.

Lesson: By asking for it in writing, the doctor has said no without saying no. He has also given himself time to consider the offer after receiving additional information.

As a busy physician, colleagues and others constantly request you to take on more projects and work. You should develop a typewritten list of 10 gentle excuses that you can keep on your desk and in your wallet so you can politely decline most of these requests. This list can and will save you hundreds of hours per year. Make your list and pull it out as soon as you hear the words, "Doctor, will you be able to...?" The authors have placed 10 sample responses in Box 2.3.

Box 2.3

Polite Ways to Say No

1. I would love to, but my plate is full.
2. That sounds great, but I'm swamped.
3. I am honored, but I'm now focusing on other areas.
4. Sounds interesting, could you please send me a written proposal?
5. I think I understand what you're looking for. I'm going to refer you to my colleague, Doctor Swensen; he is the real guru in that area.
6. Let me check my travel schedule and get back to you.
7. I'm sorry, but I have a previous family commitment. I'm (planning a wedding, caring for an elderly parent, traveling to a graduation, moving a daughter to college, etc.).

8. I can't. Ever since my (insert medical condition such as hypertension) was diagnosed, I'm under strict orders from *my* doctor not to take on any additional work.

9. I wish I could, but I'm so busy now that I'm just trying to keep my head above water.

10. I'm sorry, but that's out of the question. I've been out of the office and I'm just trying to dig out here.

Example 2.18

Q: You are a forty-five-year-old physician with a busy forensic and consulting practice who lives in New England. You have been requested to give a keynote lecture in Australia. The organization will pay for your airfare. You end up staying two weeks on vacation with your spouse. How much has this "free" trip cost you?

A: Two weeks lost income: $10,000
Spouse's airfare: $1,000
Hotel: $2,800
Meals: $2,000

Lesson: Your "free" airline ticket cost you $15,800. You may have been better off just saying no.

Chapter 3 The Best Place to Negotiate

The Home Field Advantage

The conventional wisdom expressed by most negotiation experts is that negotiators are best served by holding the negotiation session in their own office. The sports analogy of the home field advantage is used to explain why negotiations should take place in one's own office. The home team feels more comfortable, is well rested, is eating and sleeping at home, and has not been worn down by travel. In addition, when you negotiate on your own turf you have access to your files, documents, reference materials, computers, copiers, and fax machines. You can also control the logistics of the negotiation, including seating, temperature, refreshments, and to some extent, interruptions. It is also more economical because you do not incur travel costs or miss additional time from the office due to travel.

The problem with this conventional wisdom from a physician's standpoint is that each advantage listed above can be a distinct and serious disadvantage as well. See Example 3.1.

Example 3.1
Opponent: Doctor, will you be able to provide 401(k) plans for all of your employees?
Doctor: I don't know. It will be a question of finances. I will have to look into it and get back to you in a few weeks.

Opponent: Well, doctor, it's good we are in your office because all the information we need is at our fingertips. There's your bookkeeper. Let's run the numbers on Quicken and do some spreadsheets to see what you can realistically afford.

Lesson: The "advantage" of the physician negotiating on her home turf has quickly turned into a disadvantage.

Home Field Disadvantage

The disadvantages of physicians negotiating in their own offices are substantial.

INTERRUPTIONS

If you negotiate in your own office you could be subject to constant interruptions, phone calls, or noise from fax machines, computers, printers, staff, patients, and all the other distractions that come with a busy medical practice. This can make it difficult to concentrate and focus on the negotiation at hand. Under a situation such as this, you could become tempted to just get the negotiation over with so you can get back to work. Such thinking could cost you a lot of money.

UNWANTED DISCLOSURE OF INFORMATION

Inviting your opponent into your office means that he or she can view your operation, talk to your staff and patients, view your facilities, and see how much reading material is piled up on and around your desk. The information your opponents can gather from simply sitting in your waiting room for 15 minutes may provide them with powerful tools that they can use against you during the negotiation.

Example 3.2

Background: A physician is negotiating the sale of his solo practice. He has invited a prospective purchaser to his office to negotiate terms, especially the price. The purchaser arrives 30 minutes early (always a good idea) and takes a seat in the waiting room. The doctor is busy seeing patients.

Opponent: (to patient in your waiting room) How do you like the doctor and staff?

Patient: Well, the doctor herself is a great doctor, but it takes three weeks to get an appointment. I almost always see the nurse practitioner and the billing system is often inaccurate. Let me tell you what happened to my friend Pam last week....

Lesson: Important information has been revealed. It is likely that the purchaser will offer less money to the selling physician.

Deflecting Decisions

As we have seen in Example 3.1, in your own office, due to the availability of your records, staff, computer, and partners, it is more difficult to use lack of information (see pages 39-82 and 122-126 on information) as an excuse to postpone or deflect a decision. This inability to delay a decision can be a distinct disadvantage. This is particularly so when time is on your side.

Example 3.3

Background: You are part of a four-person practice and have been approached to sell your practice to a large corporation. You are appointed by your three partners to meet with the buyer at the group's office.

Opponent: We can offer you $500,000 cash and 25,000 shares of unrestricted HealthCo common stock (series A).

Doctor: I need to sit down with my partners and discuss this. We'll get back to you after we discuss it.

Opponent: I just flew in from the West Coast and don't want to have to fly here again. Why don't you discuss it with them now, while we're all in the same building? I'll wait here and you can let me know in an hour or so....

Lesson: It may be harder to delay a decision or deflect a question if you are negotiating in your own office.

LOGISTICS

Having someone come to your office to negotiate will mean that you or your staff will have to clean up and be concerned with refreshments, lunch, making photocopies, and providing support material and staff. It is not uncommon for one or two copies to turn into hours of extra work for your staff. You may want to consider the staff time and office disruption involved in having a negotiation at your office.

PREPARATION AND FOCUS

Negotiating in your own office may result in you preparing inadequately. (See pages 117-132 on preparation.) For example, you may be less inclined to focus on organizing your materials, files, and research before the negotiation. When they know they are going to a negotiation off-site, physicians tend to prepare all the materials they need and spend more time getting organized. Even more importantly, when you negotiate off site, it is natural for you to focus more on the negotiation at hand because you are removed from the distractions of your own office.

AUTHORS' RECOMMENDATION

Physicians are not necessarily best served by negotiating in their own offices. Physicians should strive to negotiate in the location that feels most comfortable, offers them the most advantages, and has the fewest drawbacks. Frequently, it is best for physicians to negotiate in neutral locations or at the offices of their opponents. In this way, you can become and remain focused on your negotiation and can learn valuable information about your opponents without being subjected to interruptions, distractions, and the unwanted disclosure of information. In short, you can prepare and concentrate on the matters under negotiation. Remember, "You don't get what you deserve. You get what you negotiate."[1]

---

[1] Chester L. Karrass

Chapter 4 Controlling and Obtaining Information

One of the key elements of any negotiation is information. Understanding how to get information from your opponent and how to prevent the disclosure of harmful information to your opponent is crucial for your development as a successful physician negotiator.

Authority

The first piece of information you will need to determine quickly is the authority of your opponent. By *authority* we mean the ability or power to say yes, to compromise on crucial terms, and to enter into a binding agreement. You should negotiate with a "yes person," a person who has the ability to agree and make things happen. The first order of business, therefore, *before* you start to negotiate, is to determine if you are negotiating with the right person. You need to determine if the person you are dealing with has the authority to negotiate and close the deal.

Example 4.1
Doctor: As you know, we have four items we need to finalize an agreement on today.
Opponent: Let me write down your needs. I will talk to my superiors and get back to you next week.
Doctor: Thank you very much for your offer to convey a message for me, but I need to deal directly with the decision makers. Let's set up a time when I can talk to them directly.

Lesson: The doctor was told up front that his opponent did not have the authority to close a deal. The doctor recognized that he could not gain anything by talking to the powerless information gatherer and correctly demanded to talk to the decision makers. Note how this demand was made in a polite way designed not to alienate the opponent's subordinate.

If the person you are dealing with is not the person with authority, find out who is. There are several methods to do this. The simplest and most direct method is to ask your opponent, "Do you have the authority to negotiate and finalize the deal *today*?" Anything less than a direct *yes* means your opponent does not have complete and unfettered authority and will have to obtain approval of any proposed deal by a third party or parties, usually at a later date. This person is usually just gathering information and feeling you out at your expense. When confronted with this situation, you can respond as in Example 4.2.

Example 4.2
Doctor: As I understand it, you are merely on a fact-finding mission here today. Who has the authority to authorize compromises and concessions so we can finalize this agreement?

Lesson: You may need to directly ask your opponent who has the full authority.

It is also helpful for you to determine in advance your opponent's decision-making process or procedure and the time frame in which decisions are normally made. You will need this information so that you can plan on when a deal will be closed or when you will have to proceed to an alternative plan if the deal can't be consummated. (See pages 117-132 on preparation.) Consider Example 4.3.

Example 4.3

Doctor: I am calling to confirm our meeting on Friday at 1:00 P.M., in your office, to negotiate the proposed contract.

Opponent: That's correct. Park in the B lot and take elevator #3 directly to the 26th floor.

Doctor: What is the procedure your company uses to finalize these types of contracts? What is your time frame?

Opponent: I will finalize an agreement and, subject to the approval of my supervisor, we will be all set. I have never had an agreement turned down yet. I am shooting for next Monday to wrap this whole deal up.

Lesson: The physician negotiator has determined the scope of his opponent's authority and has a fairly firm time line as to when he will get a final yes or no. If the answer is no, he can make alternative arrangements.

The successful physician negotiator should negotiate directly with a person who has full authority because:

1. it is easier to obtain major concessions from this person (subordinates are unsure of what the boss might think),
2. it avoids delay (there is no need to run it up the flagpole),

3. you avoid bargaining against yourself (never a good idea), and

4. you avoid the trickle-down loss on key points (see page 44 on trickle-down loss).

CONCESSIONS

If the person you are negotiating with has full authority, he or she can make concessions without having to obtain approval from anyone else. Frequently, this is done to close the deal (see pages 257-268 on closing the deal) or as a response to some concessions you have made (see pages 139-148 on concessions). Without this authority, the spontaneity of the negotiation process is lost and you will run the risk of negotiating against yourself.

DELAY

If the person does not have full authority, key concessions and compromises will have to be run up the flagpole. This means a delay and a break in the negotiation process. A break in the momentum can sometimes increase the difficulty of ultimately achieving an agreement. In addition, it will certainly increase the amount of time and effort you will need to spend on the negotiation. You should therefore always strive to negotiate with a person with full authority.

Example 4.4
You are running a little late for a short meeting with Dr. Lin at the hospital. You pull into the visitors' parking lot and it is full. The only remaining spots are for staff. You ask the security person at the lot if you could leave the car for 30 minutes, explaining your predicament. She says yes. This is an example of negotiating with

the "yes person." This person has the authority to let you park in the spot. You obtain a quick response to your request because it does not need approval from a higher authority. What if you had called Dr. Lin on your car phone? Would the result have been as effective? What if you had not talked to the security person? Would you have been more or less likely to be towed?

BARGAINING AGAINST YOURSELF

Negotiating with a person without full authority will result in the error of bargaining against yourself. When you bargain against yourself, your opponent can extract your bottom line from you and you will gain nothing in return. You will then be turned over to a person with full authority to start the negotiation process in earnest.

Example 4.5
Proposed employer: As I understand it, you want $150,000 but would accept $140,000 and you are willing to be on call occasionally.
Doctor: I am trying to be honest and fair.
Proposed employer: Let me get the administrator in on this as she is the one with the ultimate authority.
Administrator: I see you are looking for $140,000 and can work on call when needed. We can offer you $130,000 and will need you every other weekend and one night per week.

Lesson: In the above example, the employer was able to gain substantial concessions from the physician regarding salary and call while the physician gained nothing in return. Bargaining against yourself should be avoided whenever possible.

TRICKLE-DOWN LOSS

The successful physician negotiator understands and avoids *trickle-down loss*. To explain what we mean by trickle-down loss, let's suppose that you are negotiating with a company to sell them a new medical device you invented to take splinters out of someone's finger. The CEO decides that she can pay a 5% production royalty. She so instructs the department manager. He wants to look good, so he tells the legal department to offer you 4%. The attorney negotiating with you has authority at 4 %. He also wants to look good, so he offers you 3% "firm." This is the trickle-down loss in operation. Every time the terms have gone through a person's hands has cost you money. Thus, to save money, you need to negotiate with a person as high up the chain of authority as possible.

YOUR OWN AUTHORITY

You also need to be concerned with the extent of your own authority. When you are negotiating for yourself, your practice, or even your partners, your opponent will want to find out whether or not *you* have full authority. If you do have full authority, you are in a dangerous position. When you have full authority, by definition you will be able to make quick decisions and concessions without consulting anyone and without thinking them through fully.

Example 4.6
Salesperson: You have looked at the equipment three times. We met your price of $27,000 and your payment terms. You do have the authority to purchase the equipment, don't you?
Doctor: Yes, of course. It is my practice.

Salesperson: Great! Here's the contract. Please sign on pages 4, 10, and 15.

Lesson: It is frequently in your best interest to not have complete authority to negotiate and finalize agreements. If you don't have full authority, or if you profess to have limited authority, it will be easier for you to negotiate slowly and deliberately and to continue to look for better terms before agreeing to a deal. Some good ways to profess to have limited authority are listed in Box 4.1.

Box 4.1

Ways to Profess Limited Authority
1. I will have to check with my partner, supervisor, spouse, lawyer, accountant, tax advisor, etc. (who is unavailable). 2. I have another deal pending. Finalizing this agreement depends upon my successfully completing the previous deal. 3. I will have to check to see if this creates any conflicts of interest for me. 4. I want to avoid even the appearance of impropriety.

Intentionally limiting your own authority when negotiating is an excellent strategy. Savvy physician negotiators understand how to use their own lack of authority as an offensive tactic. By intentionally limiting your own authority, you can avoid making a quick agreement that has not been methodically evaluated. It will also help stop you from being pressured into deals you are not sure of and will help you overcome any tendencies you might have to "give away the store."

Example 4.7

Salesperson: This is our best offer: $27,000 for the computer equipment and one year of service.

Doctor: Our partnership agreement prevents me from signing any contracts in excess of $25,000 without the written approval of my 14 partners. The next time we will be having a full board meeting is three months from now. I can try and put this on the agenda and hopefully we can get to it at that time. If we don't get to it then....

Salesperson: If I take $2,000 out of my commission and cut the price back to $25,000, will you sign the contract today?

Doctor: Let me see the contract, please....

Lesson: The doctor cleverly uses his professed lack of authority to extract a concession of 7.4% ($2,000) off the seller's "best" offer.

Example 4.8

Q: You are negotiating the sale of your four-physician practice. The potential buyer makes a serious and fair offer to you and is pressing for a decision on the spot. What can you say to her to buy time without jeopardizing the offer?

A: One response is, "I'm going to need a couple of days to consider your proposal. Let me talk to my husband and partners and I'll get back to you in a couple of days."

Lesson: During the two-day delay you can talk things over with others and, more importantly, take the time necessary to consider the proposal.

Example 4.9
Q: You are negotiating your employment contract with a group practice. You have been contacted by the business manager to sit down and "hammer out the terms." What should you consider doing before agreeing to this meeting? Why?
A: Find out whether the business manager has full authority to bind the group. If she doesn't, politely request (and insist on, if need be) a meeting with a person in the group who does have full authority. You need to avoid negotiating against yourself and the trickle-down effect. Be prepared to respond, "I'll have to check with my spouse...." This will give you time to carefully consider the proposed agreement.

Example 4.10
Q: A managed-care company wants to come to your office and negotiate your contract with them. They will be sending their representative. What action steps could you take to control the setting and the negotiation process?
A: Make sure your partners are unavailable so that you can claim lack of full authority. Consider whether you want to change the location of the meeting to their office or a neutral location (e.g., your private club where you can wine and dine them). Verify that the representative has full authority to make changes to their contract. If not, suggest that you travel to his or her office to meet with someone who does have full authority. If you meet with a representative without full authority, use the meeting solely to extract information from that person. Do not disclose any information or negotiate against yourself.

Once you have determined the extent of your opponent's authority, you will need to determine other information about her. This information includes her needs, desires, interests, deadlines, pressures, and motives. Such information is best obtained by asking questions, using active listening skills, and by observing body language.

Asking Questions

The key to gathering information successfully in a negotiation session is to obtain as much information as possible as quickly as possible. At the same time, you want to reveal minimal key confidential information. The simplest, most direct, and most efficient method of gathering information in a negotiation session is to ask the right question at the right time. Physicians are often reluctant to ask questions that may be considered personal, impertinent, or too aggressive. It is important for you to remember that there are very important benefits to asking questions during a negotiation session. Asking good questions will help you discover key information quickly and can help you control the negotiation session flow and momentum. In addition, asking questions might be the only way to obtain certain pieces of information.

You should start the negotiation session with general, open-ended, broad questions. These will help you elicit a good deal of information right away. Open-ended questions encourage your opponent to open up and talk about his or her job, work, program, or product.

It is important for you to be a student of human nature to be a successful physician negotiator. You need to appreciate that, generally speaking, people like to talk about themselves and show how much they know about a particular subject. The more they talk, the more information they are giving you. This is a technique that the authors have used very successfully when taking depositions.

Example 4.11
Background: You have been offered a job at a group medical practice. After the head physician gives you your offer and excuses himself, you have a private chat with the office manager as you head back to your car.

Q: How do you think I should respond to the job offer?
A: Well, the offer is solid, the salary is competitive, and the fringes are okay. Now the personalities of the physicians, that is another thing....

Lesson: By asking an open-ended question, you tapped into the office manager's natural desire to help and show how much he knows. You were able to find out key information that might not have been obtainable through another source.

Another way to gain valuable information is to appear to be ignorant of certain matters. People love to teach and show off their knowledge. Let them. As one expert puts it:

> In negotiation, dumb is often better than smart, inarticulate better than articulate, and many times weakness can actually be strength. So train yourself occasionally to say, "I don't know," "I just don't understand," "You lost me some time ago," "Help me," when these phrases suit your purposes....
> Moral: Don't be too quick to "understand" or prove

your intellect at the outset of an encounter. Watch
your listen-talk ratio. Learn to ask questions even
when you think you know the answers.[1]

Understandably, this tactic is often difficult for
physicians to master. You don't often hear a doctor
say, "I don't understand" or "Help me." You should
not feel ashamed to use this technique. As trial
lawyers, the authors often had to master technical areas
that were beyond our training and scope of expertise.
We were able to do so because we were not afraid or
embarrassed to ask for help from someone with more
knowledge than ourselves, such as our expert witnesses.
You will need to develop the same attitude if you would
like to be a successful physician negotiator.

Example 4.12
Background: You have been asked to write a
screenplay for a movie about the inner workings of a
hospital. You have been offered 10% of the profits.
This is the first time you have been offered
compensation for your creative writing.

Opponent: We can offer you 10% of the profits.
Doctor: I'm sorry, I'm kind of new at this, what
exactly do you mean by profits?
Opponent: Well the accountants figure that out.
Doctor: Well, do you know how it works?
Opponent: On a basic level, sure.
Doctor: Could you explain it to me?
Opponent: Sure, you take the total revenue generated
from the movie and subtract out the expenses.
Doctor: What are the expenses?

---

[1] Cohen, 40, 42, 43.

Opponent: Production costs, distribution, allocated overhead, and some others.
Doctor: How are the production costs calculated?

Lesson: By asking questions indicating that he was not an expert in film contracts, the doctor was able to gain valuable information concerning the value of the offered contract. Had he been uncomfortable doing this, he never would have learned that by the time all the expenses have been taken out, 10% of profits could and often does amount to 10% of nothing.

After you have obtained as much information as possible by using general questions, it is best to move into more specific, pointed questions. These specific questions are most effectively asked once you have determined the exact information you need. For example, if an employer was worried about call coverage, she could simply ask, "If we were able to offer you this position, would you be willing to work one night a week and one weekend per month?"

One of the reasons for starting with general questions and moving to specific ones is that your opponent is likely to answer the general questions more freely. This is true because it is less likely that he feels that he is being led or prodded. You need to keep in mind that once you start asking specific questions your opponent is more likely to be on guard and to be more careful about his or her response.

One technique you can use to take advantage of the above-described phenomenon is to dispense with the pleasantries and easy open-ended questions and ask your most difficult pointed question at the start of the negotiation. This will often catch your opponent off guard. Your opponent is probably expecting general open-ended questions and may be unprepared to answer the "hard question" in a deceptive way. The authors call this technique "the Brooklyn approach."[2]

Example 4.13
Doctor: We are both very busy professionals. Let's cut to the chase. How much money are you offering?
Opponent: Well, I have authority to offer up to $2.5 million.

Lesson: This is the Brooklyn approach. A direct question will sometimes catch your opponent off guard and make him reveal valuable information.

To employ the Brooklyn approach, you as a physician will have to overcome any aversion you have to asking direct, pointed, and possibly difficult questions. To soften the blow to your opponent you can always follow up your question with a statement such as, "I apologize for being so direct, but I don't have any time to waste on preliminaries."

Four additional types of questions for gathering information are leading questions, suggestive questions, successive questions, and "what if" questions. *Leading questions* are questions in which statements of fact are turned into questions that contain the essence of the answer you are seeking. This type of question permits the proponent of the question to maintain control over the information flow, the momentum, and the negotiation itself. Leading questions are typically used by attorneys during cross-examination. The problem with leading questions is that they can sometimes be

---

[2] Mr. Babitsky being brought up in that borough.

offensive. Furthermore, they do not produce much information that you don't already know or suspect. Leading questions typically must be answered with a yes or a no. They can be particularly useful in pinning a person down on a point by making it much more difficult for them to be evasive. Some sample leading questions are provided in Box 4.2.

Box 4.2

Sample Leading Questions
Q: She has already exceeded her budget, hasn't she? **Q:** You are looking for a three-year agreement, correct? **Q:** You don't have a problem with..., do you? **Q:** Isn't it a fact that you have no other offers outstanding? **Q:** Isn't it true that you don't have complete authority to close this deal? **Q:** You do have some flexibility on the price, don't you?

Suggestive questions are questions that contain a suggestive course of action. These can also be useful during a negotiation. The best suggestive questions give your opponent limited choices and make it awkward for him or her to raise a third option. For example, you could ask, "Would X work better for you or Y?" As long as both of the proposed alternatives are favorable to your position, the suggestive question is a good method of obtaining closure on a particular point during the negotiation process.

Asking a series of *successive questions* can also be useful. The series of questions should point to a logical conclusion. This technique is often used by trial attorneys and is useful in controlling the negotiation process and building momentum toward your ultimate goals.

Example 4.14
Background: A doctor works for a group practice and is seeking a raise.

Doctor: Haven't I been an excellent employee?
Opponent: Sure.
Doctor: Don't my patients love me?
Opponent: The feedback has been tremendously positive.
Doctor: I am among the top three income producers in the practice, am I not?
Opponent: This year, yes.
Doctor: Who was the person who picked up the slack when Dr. Jones was out on maternity leave?
Opponent: We appreciate you pitching in.

Lesson: The successive questions lead to the inescapable conclusion that the physician is entitled to a raise!

"What if" questions can also be useful. These questions are trial balloons in which you elicit responses to less than concrete proposals or suggestions. These questions have the added advantage that they are generally not adversarial in nature.

Example 4.15
Doctor: What if we were able to offer you flex time? Would that help you?

Prospective employee: Yes, if I could make my own hours the salary could work.

Lesson: The doctor has gained valuable information without committing herself to anything.

How you ask your question can be of crucial importance. For example, let's say that you are trying to get a quick read on how firm a price really is. You could ask, "Is that price firm?" As you might expect, almost uniformly the reply will be the same—"Yes." Why is that? Because you have made it too easy for the person to turn you down. What if you asked the question a little differently? "Do you have any flexibility in the price?" Again, it is too easy to say no, and that is what you will probably hear. What if you asked the question as follows? "How much flexibility do you have in the price?" The most common response is, "Not too much." This is a lot better than no and it opens up the matter of the price. From there you are up and running and can discuss how much is "not too much."

In the course of thousands of negotiations, the authors have asked one simple question—"How much flexibility do you have?"—many times. The majority of the time the answers have been very helpful: "a little," "some," "not too much," "quite a bit." When you obtain any of these responses, the door has been opened and you can begin to negotiate the final terms. In the rare case in which the answer was "none at all" you have still gleaned important information quickly. If your opponent is being forthcoming, you may not be able to reach an agreement. Successful physician negotiators cannot be timid or afraid of asking these types of questions in this kind of way.

Asking the right questions during a negotiation is an art as much as it is a science.[3] How to properly

---

[3] As an art, we can learn a lot from studying the "masters." McCormack lists the five questions that need to be answered during the negotiation:

> What, When, Where, How Exclusive, and How Much? All five of the questions asked above should be answered during the course of negotiation.
> A. The What
> What is it, precisely, that you are selling?
> B. The When
> This means how long, from "one contiguous eight-hour period," which can be used to define a workday, to "forever."
> C. The Where
> "Territory," which can range from "the world" to "South Cincinnati."
> D. The How Exclusive
> To what degree does the buyer wish (and are we willing) to shut out the rest of the competition?
> E. The How Much
> This means money, but not necessarily money alone. It can also mean stocks, securities, or other forms of equity.

Mark H. McCormack, *What They Don't Teach You at Harvard Business School: Notes from a Street Smart Executive* (New York: Bantam Books, 1984) 142–144.

Donaldson lists handy guidelines for asking better questions during a negotiation:

> • Plan your questions in advance.
> • Ask with a purpose.
> • Tailor your question to your listener.
> • Follow general questions with more specific ones.
> • Keep questions short and clear. Cover only one subject.
> • Make transitions between their answers and your questions.

respond to your opponent's questions is equally, if not more, important.

Answering Questions

When you use questions effectively, you can expect that your opponent will ask you a series of questions as well. How you respond to these questions is as much an art as knowing which questions to ask. "The art of answering questions in negotiation lies in knowing what to answer and what not to; when to be clear and when not to. It does not lie in being right or wrong."[4]

It is important that you not let your training as a physician influence the way you respond to questions. You have been trained to respond to queries with complete, responsive answers. As a physician negotiator you should remember that *just because your opponent asks you a question does not mean that you have to answer it or answer it fully.*

When answering questions, keep your answers as short as possible. Don't volunteer information. Do make sure that you do not disclose any confidential information. Preparation and planning are extremely important if you want to be able to deal effectively with difficult questions. As part of your preparation you need to decide what information you will disclose and under what circumstances you will disclose it. You need to weigh how the disclosure of information will assist the negotiation process or impede it. You will

---

• Don't interrupt. Let the other person answer the question.
• Avoid leading questions.
Michael C. Donaldson and Mimi Donaldson, *Negotiating for Dummies* (Chicago: IDG Books Worldwide, 1996) 138, 139.
[4] Chester L. Karrass, *The Negotiating Game* (New York: Harper Business, Revised Edition, 1992) 193.

also need to judge how much the disclosure or nondisclosure of information will affect your credibility and integrity in the eyes of your opponent.

When dealing with difficult questions, you should remember the four D's: deferring, deflecting, delaying, or declining to answer the question. These are the techniques that are used by politicians when responding (or, more appropriately, *not* responding) to difficult, pointed questions. Note that none of the responses involve untruths. Examples of the four D's are given in Box 4.3.

Box 4.3

The Four D Methods
Defer: "That's an excellent question. Let's hold that for now and get back to it after we have some more information." *Deflect:* "I appreciate your concern. What I am worried about is...." *Delay:* "That question gets to the heart of the problem. I need some time to think that over." *Decline:* "I don't know" *(or)* "Let me look into it."[5]

---

[5] For additional declining techniques in highly sensitive areas you can:

- rule the question out of bounds as improper or inappropriate,
- ignore the apparent inquiry,
- answer a different question,
- answer only the beneficial part of a complex question,
- respond generally to a specific inquiry, or
- respond specifically to a general inquiry.

Charles B. Craver, *Effective Legal Negotiation and Settlement* (Massachusetts Continuing Legal Education, Inc., 1996) 23.

Ilich suggests some other techniques that you can use to deal with difficult questions. These techniques are provided for you in Box 4.4.

Box 4.4

More Techniques to Deal with Difficult Questions

Plead ignorance: "I just don't know" *(or)* "I'm not familiar with that."
Plead irrelevance: "That's irrelevant" *(or)* "That's not important. What *is* important is...."
Personal: "That's just too personal, I'm not going to get into that area."
Answer with a question: "I haven't determined that yet. How much are *you* looking for?"[6]

Some early questions can be in writing. Sometimes, before negotiation starts, we will ask our opponents to send us a one- or two-page memo telling us:

1. what their goals and objectives are, and
2. how they propose we work together to meet these objectives.

The detailed answers that we get are remarkable. These then can set the tone for the entire negotiation. They let us know "where they are coming from" before we even get to the negotiation table. This technique is particularly useful in screening out potential deals where the opponent has nothing of real benefit to offer. Negotiating is time consuming and you

---

[6]John Ilich, *The Complete Idiot's Guide to Winning through Negotiation* (New York: Alpha Books, 1996) 69.

should not waste your time on a potential deal unless your opponent has something of value to offer you.

Example 4.16

Q: You are the physician owner of a series of health clinics. While flying to the West Coast you meet a mergers and acquisitions expert who says he can make you a lot of money and help you "cash out" of your business. You get very excited and agree to fly to Seattle (from New York) the following week to discuss details. What have you done wrong?

A: 1. Your excitement has disclosed the confidential information that you are over-eager to sell. This will be very detrimental to any terms you could obtain, especially price. 2. Before you commit the time and expense of entering into negotiations 3,000 miles from home, you need to find out where your opponent is coming from. Is he interested in buying you out via cash or stock in a high profile, publicly traded company or is he offering stock in a start up company (which could be next to worthless)? This question should be asked up front.

As a successful physician negotiator, you need to obtain crucial information from your opponent quickly and efficiently. This can be done by asking the right questions at the right time, in the manner most likely to result in a complete and accurate response. At the same time, you need to closely guard your confidential information and defer, deflect, delay, and decline to answer difficult questions that could harm you.

Example 4.17

Q: You are the managing partner of a six-person orthopedic practice in Longview, Texas. On January 4, 1998, at 5:00 P.M., a twenty-five-year-old law student, Jamie Curtis, tripped over a parking divider in your parking lot and sustained a fractured ankle (posterior malleolus). She was treated by your office by reduction and fixation, physical therapy, and had a walking cast for three months. She has made a good recovery. She incurred medical expenses of $4,950 of which $4,250 was paid for by her health insurer. You will be meeting Ms. Curtis in five minutes to discuss "settling" her claim against your office for inadequate lighting in your parking lot. Ms. Curtis has some residual stiffness on rainy days and says if the matter is not settled today, she will retain her uncle, Gerry Spence, to represent her. Your office manager let your general liability policy lapse without renewing it on December 3, 1997. You have no insurance coverage for this accident. You have consulted with your attorney, who would be pleased to defend your group for $250 per hour with a $15,000 retainer. He tells you that you have a 40% chance of winning at trial. He estimates that defense costs would run between $15,000 and $25,000. If the case were lost, a judgment would likely be between $45,000 and $125,000 depending on how things "break" at the trial. He mailed you a blank "full and final release form" and urged you not to try and resolve this yourself. You feel that Ms. Curtis appreciates the excellent medical care she was given and will be reasonable. Your partners, after blaming you for not having insurance coverage, asked you to settle the case as quickly and as cheaply as possible. Ms. Curtis has thirty minutes to meet with you before she has to get to her class on medical malpractice. In the spirit of negotiation, she has agreed to answer your questions. What will you ask her and why?

A: You need to find out very quickly what this woman is looking for. Is she just looking for her $700.00 in unpaid medical expenses? She's a law student. She probably has a very good idea what her claim is worth if she pushes it. The crucial question is, does she want to push it? After this trip and fall she was treated by your office. You think she is satisfied. The authors would start this negotiation with pleasantries and ask her how she is doing. You need to get a read on her desires and motives. Look for body language and tone. Is this woman looking for a pound of flesh? They would then apologize for any pain that she has been in and tell her how much they've enjoyed helping her get better. We want her to like us and to keep this from turning into an adversarial situation. We would then ask if there was anything we could do to help her recover financially from this tragic accident and ask her about the $700.00 insurance deficiency. If all she is looking for is the $700.00, that is all the doctor should offer. (The doctor should also mention to this law student that the group has no insurance for this claim. She'll then understand that the offer is from the group's pocket and that if she pushed her claim, that any money would come out of the group's pocket as well.)

Example 4.18

Q: Joseph Stevens, M.D., age 34, is an internist and is interested in joining a professional corporation of physicians, Falmouth Associates, Inc., in his hometown of Falmouth, Massachusetts. Dr. Stevens is licensed in both Massachusetts and Connecticut. Falmouth, Massachusetts is a rural community on Cape Cod with 35,000 year-round residents and 500,000 summer visitors. It has one hospital, the Falmouth Hospital, and has affiliations with the Cape Cod Hospital twenty-five miles away and Massachusetts General Hospital seventy-five miles to the north. Falmouth Associates, Inc., is one of only two groups of internists in Falmouth, Massachusetts. Joseph Stevens, M.D., is Board Certified and Falmouth Associates, Inc., is well thought of in the community. The average salary for internists nationwide is $174,000. The average salary for internists in rural areas is $124,000. Falmouth Associates, Inc., has four full-time physicians, ages forty-nine, fifty-four, fifty-six, and sixty-three, who are all partners. It also has two physician assistants, ages forty-four and fifty-three, and a support staff of twelve. The clinic has 4,500 patients in Falmouth and the surrounding area. You, as managing partner, are extremely busy and your staff and partners work long hours. Each partner is on call three nights a week and one weekend per month. The partners are earning $259,000 per year but are complaining bitterly about the toll the long hours are taking on them, their health, and their families. You have had to turn away new patients and have a long waiting time for patients to get an appointment. You are concerned about hiring a "local" because he may quit the practice and go out on his own. You want someone willing to work hard. You feel that you must hire a good internist quickly. You do not mind training a new doctor as long as he or she will be a team player and stay with the practice. Due to the rural nature of Falmouth, it is hard to get high quality young doctors. Your partners were impressed with the CV of Dr. Stevens and have told you in no uncertain terms that if you do not hire him, they will be very upset and may want to break up the practice and go to work elsewhere. As you were leaving, they also said, "Make sure you don't give away the store." What questions will you ask him at the beginning of the negotiation? What other questions might you ask him as the negotiation progresses?

A: You need to find out at the outset *how badly* this person wants to come to work in Falmouth. Is he entertaining offers from Connecticut and other parts of Massachusetts? Does he have his heart set on Falmouth? If he does have his heart set on Falmouth (his hometown), you may be able to hire him for much less money than otherwise because there is only one other group of internists in Falmouth. You will also need to find out his willingness to be a team player, work hard, and take call. Note that any deal you strike will need to contain a covenant not to compete that will protect the practice.

Active Listening

To gather as much information as possible, the successful physician negotiator needs to develop active listening skills.[7] Through using active listening skills

---

[7] "The ability to listen, really to hear what someone is saying has far greater business implications, of course, than simply gaining insight into people.... The bottom line is that almost any business situation will be handled differently, and with different results, by someone who is listening and someone who isn't." Mark H. McCormack, *What They Don't Teach You at Harvard Business School: Notes from a Street Smart Executive* (New York: Bantam Books, 1984) 8.

"The need for listening is obvious yet is difficult to do; listen well, listening enables you to understand their perceptions, feel their emotions, and hear what they are trying to say. Active listening improves not only what you hear, but also what they say." Roger Fisher and William Ury (Bruce Patton, ed.), *Getting to Yes: Negotiating Agreement without Giving In* (New York: Penguin, 1991) 34.

you can often obtain the information that you need. In a negotiation your opponent might not repeat the key information. Frequently, physicians and many other professionals ask questions and do not listen to the answers. This happens because the physician is fiddling with papers, being interrupted by phone calls, pagers, or is thinking of something else. Prior to negotiating, you should clear your desk and instruct your staff not to allow any interruption. Consider Box 4.5.

Box 4.5

Five Key Active Listening Mistakes

1. Anticipating or assuming (even worse) what the opponent will say.
2. Finishing the opponent's sentences.
3. Thinking about or starting the next question.
4. Trying to impress the opponent or other parties participating in the negotiation with your general intelligence or grasp of the topic.
5. Second-guessing the statements being made.

The three specific active listening skills you need to develop to be a successful physician negotiator are the ability to hear all that is said, the ability to hear what is omitted, and the ability to listen and hear equivocal statements and verbal leaks.

When you as a physician negotiator are presented with a request, demand, or statement that will affect the negotiation, you need to hear it fully. You also need to understand what your opponent means. Do

---

"Active listening is more difficult than most people realize.... You must be alert to listen.... Active listening involves all the senses and many listening devices." Donaldson and Donaldson, 118.

not be too proud to ask for a clarification of a term that is vague, that is technical, that you might not understand, or that your opponent *may* be giving a different meaning to than you are.

Example 4.19
Educational provider: Doctor, we would like you to develop a high quality two-day educational program.
Doctor: When you say "high quality," what do you mean specifically? I want to make sure we are on the same page before we talk cost.

Lesson: The physician negotiator is clarifying what his opponent means. He is not *assuming* that he knows what is meant by the term "high quality." The details of a deal and what is meant by certain terms are critical. It is important for you not to agree to something before you know—in no ambiguous terms—what the details are.

Example 4.20
Publisher: Because you are the world's leading expert on impairment and disability, we would like you to do "the" book for us.
Doctor: Great! When do you need the book finished by?

Lesson: Now the doctor cannot negotiate effectively about price, compensation, editorial help, marketing, or budget. He has agreed so rapidly to a deal that any further negotiation on terms will be difficult. (See pages 261-265 on when you have an agreement.)

Example 4.21

Publisher: Doctor, because you are the world's leading expert on impairment and disability, we would like you to do "the" book for us.

Doctor: That sounds interesting. As you know, I am quite busy, but still interested. Please send me a note with the details, length, style, editorial help, compensation, advances, royalties, deadlines, etc., and I will get back to you.

Lesson: The doctor has "heard" the publisher—she wants a book. The publisher no doubt now has "heard" the doctor—she will have to work hard to get him. The author will not come cheap, but if there is a fair deal, the publisher can get the author she wants.

To prevent misunderstandings, you can paraphrase your opponent's statement and restate it in your own words. As the negotiation proceeds toward closure, these misunderstandings can lead to deadlock. (See pages 257-268 on closing.) Paraphrasing your opponent's statement will give her an opportunity to correct any false impressions that may have developed. In addition, you can condense a long, complex proposal into a short, clear statement. For example, you could say, "So, as I understand it, what you are saying is that your bottom line is $150,000 a year plus the fringes we discussed, correct?"

A similar technique you can use is to reframe your opponent's statement by putting it into a different form, size, or scope. The five reframing techniques that the successful physician negotiator should strive to master are listed in Box 4.6.

Box 4.6

Reframing Techniques
1. *Ordering:* The active listener sorts the content elements into a logical sequence based on such things as importance, size, timing, and amount.   2. *Grouping:* The active listener organizes the content elements according to common ideas and issues.   3. *Fractionating:* The active listener breaks a large and complex problem or idea into smaller parts that can be more easily understood and managed (or ordered or grouped).   4. *Expanding:* The active listener expands or elaborates on an issue or idea that is stated in generalized terms and offers it for verification for accuracy.   5. *Generalizing:* The active listener identifies the general issues or ideas, omitting the details that expand or elaborate and may confuse this general theme.[8]

It is just as important to appreciate what is *not* being said as it is to hear and understand what is being said. Consider the following example.

Example 4.22
Background: A physician and his two partners are invited to a two-hour dinner meeting with a physician in Hawaii. The Hawaiian physician spends most of the evening extolling the virtues of some new diagnostic

---

[8] U.S. Army Corps of Engineers, "When People Complain: Using Communication, Negotiation, and Problem-Solving to Resolve Complaints" (IWR Report 91-R-4, 1991) 35.

testing equipment he and others have developed. The mainland physician and his two partners were attempting to obtain a contract for help in marketing this new device. After the meeting the three partners met and debriefed each other. While two partners were discussing the terms of the marketing agreement, the other partner said, "You know, I think he is trying to get us to invest in his equipment.". The other two partners disagreed strongly. They pointed out quite correctly that the physician from Hawaii never mentioned investments or made any reference to investing any money. At a subsequent meeting, the pointed question was finally asked:

Q: Would you like us to invest in your new equipment?
A: Yes.

Lesson: The physician from Hawaii was not looking for a marketing partner or contract at all. He was looking for an investor. This true story is a good example of listening to what is *not* being said and appreciating a message that is not verbalized. A good active listener understands that what is not being verbalized is often more important than what is being said actively. This is because, many times, your opponent is trying to get you to draw your own conclusions or come up with the idea yourself. In the above example, the three partners would be more likely to invest if they concluded that this was a good idea themselves. Thus, leaving out the specific request for money was in fact intentional and an excellent strategy to solicit funds.

EQUIVOCAL STATEMENTS AND VERBAL LEAKS

Many times your opponents will, intentionally or unintentionally, tip you off as to their negotiating position or bottom line. This is done through making equivocal statements and verbal leaks. You need to be able to pick up on these.

Example 4.23

Doctor: Do you have any flexibility in the budget for my compensation package?

Employer: The hospital is not *inclined* to offer any more *at this time*.

Lesson: This equivocal statement tells you that the hospital does have flexibility. It will probably offer more money at some point if the doctor keeps negotiating.

As a successful physician negotiator you must be actively aware of all verbal leaks. Such leaks occur with regularity and must be appreciated if you are to obtain the best possible deal. Until you get an unequivocal response, such as, "Under no circumstances can we even consider more money," your opponent may in fact be saying to you, "There is more money on the table to be had." You need to listen hard enough to hear what is being said. To do this, you will need to devote your full and undivided attention to what is being said, practice your active listening skills, hear what is not being verbalized, and listen for verbal leaks and equivocal statements.

BODY LANGUAGE

You need to seek information from all available sources. One frequently overlooked source of information is body language. There is valuable information to be gleaned by interpreting behavioral cues.[9]

As a physician negotiator you need to be aware of the cues your opponent gives you. It is like being on second base in a baseball game and picking up the signs that the catcher is giving to the pitcher. It is all part of the game. Many physician negotiators do not recognize these cues either because they do not look for them or because they are distracted by something else.

Example 4.24
Doctor: Do you have any flexibility in the price?
Opponent: (small smile) No.
Doctor: That's too bad!

Lesson: During the smile, the doctor was not looking at the opponent because she was typing in her laptop. By not concentrating on what was important (the opponent's body language) the doctor missed the opportunity to obtain extremely valuable information.

The above example shows a lost opportunity. It also shows how crucial it is for you as a physician negotiator to not be distracted and to carefully observe your opponent. This is especially true when your

---

[9] "A cue is a message sent indirectly whose meaning may be ambiguous and require interpretation.... Behavioral cues are the language of the body as displayed in posture, facial expressions, eye contact, and hand gestures...." Cohen, 106.

opponent is going to give you an answer to a crucial question. You will miss most nonverbal cues if your head is buried in a computer or notepad. Only about half of what you need to know will be delivered in the words your opponents deliver. The other half will be in their body language, such as facial expressions, smiles, frowns, head nods, and crossed arms or legs.

A successful physician negotiator looks for the smallest indication of interest or disinterest in the face or actions of an opponent and uses that information successfully. Consider the following example.

Example 4.25

You are attempting to convince a prospective physician employee that he should accept a position in your group practice. You make point after point and the young physician sits there, impassive. Finally, you mention that your town has an excellent school system. The physician, for the first time, pulls out a pen and jots down "excellent school system." You pick up on this interest and explain the school system and extracurricular activities. You picked up on a cue given during a negotiation session and used it to your advantage.

When interpreting the body language of your opponent, it is important to remember that this is an imprecise science and that your opponent may be intentionally incorporating certain gestures to disguise his or her true feelings. With this in mind, several of the most common gestures and their accepted meanings are listed in Box 4.7.

Box 4.7

Gesture Meanings

Casual touching of person	Sincerity
Clearing throat often	Untruth
Closed fists	Anger
Cocking the head	Receptiveness
Crossing arms and legs	Not receptive to idea
Crossing, uncrossing legs	Impatience
Fidgeting with pen or pencil	Lack of confidence in position
Gritting one's teeth	Anger/trying to control anger
Leaning back in the chair	Confidence
Locking ankles	Resistance
Looking at watch	Impatience
Looking person in the eye	Sincerity
Mirroring body position	Telling opponent that "we are the same"
Nervous laugh	Unexpressed concerns
Open-handed expressions	Sincerity
Rolling eyes	Impatience/disbelief
Shifting eyes	Deceit
Sitting on the edge of chair	Interest in discussion
Staring	Aggressive, controlling behavior
Sudden raise in vocal pitch	Untruth
Touching one's face, collar, tie, etc.	Not telling the truth

It is equally important to be aware of and control the nonverbal messages *you* unintentionally give off during the negotiation session. You should maintain a poker face and not reveal what you are feeling or thinking.[10] If you do not, you could give valuable information to your opponent.

Example 4.26
You are negotiating with a potential purchaser of your home. Each time the purchaser asks you about your electric, sewer, or garage systems, you smile and immediately and enthusiastically respond, "Great." When you are asked how you like the neighbors, your smile disappears, you pause for a moment, and say that they're great as well. Your opponent picks up on this change of attitude and becomes worried. The sale falls through.

Lesson: By not maintaining a poker face, the physician unintentionally revealed the information that the neighbors are a potential problem. This nonverbal leak of information lost the deal.

NEEDS, INTERESTS, AND DESIRES

You must determine the needs, interests, and desires of the party you are negotiating with. This is not easy. Most physicians feel that they know or can figure out what their opponent needs and/or wants. Often, nothing could be further from the truth. Physician negotiators make a serious mistake when they assume that due to their intelligence, education, and experience they can sit in their office and figure out the needs, desires, objectives, motives, and interests of their opponents. You cannot necessarily take at face value what your

---

[10] "When you are negotiating the gestures you don't make can be as telling as those you do make.... a gasp, a flinch, or a smile can speak volumes about your position. Remember, your opponent is reading your attitude, your facial expressions and your tone of voice just as sharply as you are watching his." Ilich, 49.

opponent says he or she really wants. You will need to determine this information through research, inference, and deduction. Most importantly, you will need to determine this information as early in the negotiation process as possible.

All negotiations involve the needs or perceived needs of the person with whom you are negotiating. The noted psychologist Abraham Maslow categorized the needs of most people into a hierarchy: self-fulfillment needs, status needs, social/company needs, security/housing needs, and physical needs—water and food. The theory is that once a person satisfies the basic needs of water, food, security, and housing, he or she then aspires to the higher needs of status and self-fulfillment.

You must know and understand your opponent's needs before you can attempt satisfy them. To do this, you need to ask her what she is looking for. The entire field of marketing is based on this premise. Surveys, polls, needs assessments, questionnaires, and focus groups all are methods used by marketing professionals to determine what people need.

As a physician, you are or should be familiar with the needs of your colleagues. Physicians may look for financial security, respect, success, professional recognition, challenging work, autonomy, and the opportunity to help their patients and to make a difference. Typically, your colleagues are worried about limited or reduced incomes, failure, malpractice suits, managed care, risks, being second-guessed, and being taken advantage of. When negotiating with nonphysicians, you must determine as quickly as possible what they "need" to be successful.

Example 4.27
You are looking for a part-time receptionist to cover
your office two afternoons per week. You are about to
interview a sixty-seven-year-old woman who worked
for thirty-seven years as a legal secretary at a large law
firm. She seems like she'd be a great asset. You are
concerned, however, that she'll require too much
money or that she'll leave to find a more challenging
job. At the interview you ask her why she is applying
for the receptionist job. You find out that she is retired
and her husband, a Wall Street investment banker,
recently died. She is looking for a way to get out of the
house into an environment where she is useful and
helps people.

Lesson: You were able to hire an eminently qualified
employee at a reasonable rate because you determined
what the employee was (and was not) looking for.

After you determine the needs of the person you
will be negotiating with, you next want to determine
what she is interested in; that is, what is it that makes
the person tick? The successful physician negotiator
sincerely wants to understand her opponent's values
and what her opponent feels is important. Look for two
things: first, an insight into your opponent and second,
a method of bonding with that person. Areas to probe
gingerly include the following.

- Values: What does he or she find important?
- Family life: Children, pets, and spouse (in
  that order)
- Professional achievements: The living CV
- Art
- Films

- Hobbies
- Athletic achievements
- Volunteer work
- Travel
- The X factor

In almost every negotiation, you can find compatible interests to build upon.

Example 4.28
A physician from the South meets an attorney from Massachusetts at a conference in San Francisco. They are both looking for something to help build a business relationship and friendship on. After fifteen minutes they discover they both grew up in Brooklyn, New York, around the same time. The bond is formed. One sends another a gift "from one Brooklyn boy to another."

Lesson: The personal relationship that has been formed will be useful during negotiations.

Example 4.29
You are negotiating the sale of your practice to another physician. You are at an impasse. You know that the other physician is a devoted skier. You suggest that negotiations be reconvened in Vail, Colorado, so that everyone can be more focused.

Lesson: You will be more likely to gain concessions from your opponent when he is distracted and relaxed by his interest in skiing.

While all of us are familiar with most of the factors listed previously, the X factor merits further discussion. The X factor is that one single factor that is the driving force behind your opponent's personality. It is the answer to the question, "What makes Sammy run?" It is the single most important thing that interests or drives your opponent. If you can tap into this X factor, it will be a tremendous advantage in any negotiation.

Example 4.30
You determine that the person you are dealing with prides herself in her creativity and ingenuity. You congratulate her on her great new ideas, ask her how she got to be so creative, and ask if there is any way one can learn to be creative. Her personal needs (i.e., ego gratification and recognition of her creativity) have been satisfied. It is likely that she will be very receptive to your questions and to your negotiations.

Example 4.31
An excellent representation of discovering someone's X factor is in the movie *The Silence of the Lambs*. In the film, Hannibal Lector is incarcerated in a high security cell but demonstrates a killer's instinct for quickly getting to the heart of his opponent's personality. Clarise is the FBI agent who comes to the cell to question and match wits with him. He questions Clarise about her upbringing, her father dying when she was very young, and her going to live with an uncle on a farm. The killing and screaming of the lambs are what drove her. She could still hear it and had nightmares. Hannibal Lector got into her psyche. He found out what drove her to a position in authority.

If you can tap into your opponent's X factor—the single most important factor that drives him or her, you will know how to prepare for your negotiation sessions.

What is the object of all this psychological delving? There are five important reasons to consider psychological factors.

1. You want to create a *comfortable relationship*.
2. You want to *bond* with the other person.
3. You want to develop *trust* and *respect*.
4. You want to discover and develop *shared compatible interests*.
5. **You want the other person to like you.**

The last point is most important and cannot be overemphasized. The people you negotiate with will go to extraordinary lengths to help and assist you if they truly like you. Thus, you will get better deals and terms.

When you tap into the X factor you can often convert your opponent into an ally. If this happens, you will have found someone that is willing to go to bat for you, to work for you, to make a case for you. What you really have is a friend who is championing your position. You opponent's prestige becomes tied to the negotiation, to the deal, and sometimes even to his position in his company. He is no longer an opponent but is more like a partner. Once you are in it together and you and your opponent fight the problem, you are at least halfway there.

Example 4.32
You are negotiating with a salesperson. You start talking casually about sales quotas and determine that the quarter end is in two days. You tell the salesperson that you will do everything you can to help her meet her quota and to get her a commission.

Lesson: The salesperson appreciates your trying to help and you now know that she needs to close the deal. You can get favorable terms.

Example 4.33
You will be negotiating a lease renewal for your group's office space in a few months. Your landlord is an acquaintance whose son is very interested in professional football. You own season tickets to your local professional team. Two days before the biggest game of the year, you offer your tickets (free of charge) to the landlord. You state that "something came up" and you can't use the tickets yourself.

Lesson: By tapping into your landlord's strong desire to take care of his family, you have helped to build a very positive relationship that will be useful during your upcoming lease negotiations.

Example 4.34
Some years ago we were building a relationship and friendship with a new client. She casually mentioned one day over dinner that as a child her favorite book was *The Land of the Lost Buttons*. She wanted to show a copy to her children but was unable to find it. After returning to our office, we made an all-out effort to locate this book, which had been out of print for 35

years. It took us six months, but we finally located it. We sent the book along to her with a note that said: "The difficult we do routinely, the impossible takes a little longer." As you might expect, she was overwhelmed and will never forget our small kindness.

Example 4.35

Q: You are entering into an employment negotiation with a hospital administrator. As part of your preparation you will make a list of things that he may try to achieve with this negotiation. Name ten general things he may try to accomplish.

A:
1. Look like a hero with the Board.
2. Seek additional power.
3. Hire a team player.
4. Come in under budget.
5. Get the best qualified physician.
6. Hire someone he bonds with.
7. Hire someone who is willing to take a lot of call.
8. Hire a person with a lot of relevant experience.
9. Hire the most highly intelligent physician.
10. Hire someone with local roots.

Lesson: In preparing to negotiate, you will need to fashion responses addressing each of these potential desires of your opponent.

As a successful physician negotiator, you need to develop fully your potential for identifying the needs, interests, and desires of your opponents. You can often satisfy these needs without sacrificing your own goals. Successful physician negotiators will determine what their opponents' needs, interests, and desires are and act accordingly.

Chapter 5 The Best Time to Negotiate

Successful physician negotiators realize that timing plays a crucial part in most negotiations. In fact, timing may be everything in certain negotiations. The four key elements of timing in negotiations are: when to negotiate, when to pause, setting and dealing with the acceptance time, and the use and abuse of deadlines.

When to Negotiate

The best time to negotiate is when you need the deal the least and your opponent needs the deal or agreement the most. You must plan ahead. You should avoid having to negotiate when you desperately need a deal.[1]

Example 5.1

Q: You will be interviewing for a new position at a growing group medical practice. You have a comfortable position but would like to improve your financial situation. Your prospective employer is short two physicians and is working seven days a week to keep up with the workload. His partners have told him to hire someone *now* or they will also leave. In this example, who is negotiating at a good time?

A: The physician who seeks to improve his situation has a much stronger bargaining position. He doesn't need to accept a position. He can choose to accept it if

---

[1] Of course, if this is not possible and you are forced to negotiate, you need to avoid revealing to your opponent the fact that you are desperate to make a deal.

it meets all his requirements. The group is in a disadvantageous situation. It needs to hire someone as soon as possible. If the group tries to hold out for its best terms, it risks not hiring someone soon enough.

The time pressures that you are under in a negotiation should be clearly known to you. What you do not know, however, is what time pressures exist for your opponent. This is information that you need to determine. One technique that is frequently used to do this during out-of-town negotiations is the *flight back gambit.* Consider the following example.

Example 5.2
Q: Doctor, what time is your flight back out of O'Hare tonight?
A: 5:30 P.M. on United.
Q: Don't worry. You can leave from downtown at 4:45 P.M. and still make it.

Lesson: With this innocent sounding question, the opponent has learned the extent of the doctor's time pressure for the day's meeting. At the same time, she has gotten him thinking about the last minute, impossible race against time to O'Hare Airport. With this innocent question, the doctor has made it difficult for you to concentrate on the negotiation session.

A second time gambit consists of simply asking your opponent when she needs to close the deal. This obvious technique can be very useful in determining your opponent's time deadlines, gaining you a timing advantage. Consider the following example.

Example 5.3
Q: Doctor, when do you want to wrap this up by?
A: I need to have this tied down by Thursday.

Lesson: While this gambit might seem obvious, it is still quite efficient and of frequent use. Here the physician's opponent has learned the key timing information (when the opponent must have closure). This will clearly give the opponent the timing advantage. Note that it may be difficult for the physician to be dishonest in this situation. If he really needs a deal by Thursday, but states otherwise, the physician risks that the deal will fall through because his opponent will not feel obliged to follow up within the required period.

You need to recognize and avoid being caught in ambush negotiations. (See pages 27-31.) The ambush negotiation is one way an opponent can use the physician time pressure gambit. This gambit is used repeatedly against physicians who are often too busy to argue. Consider the following examples.

Example 5.4
Broker: Doctor, about that sailboat you and your spouse liked. We are down to crunch time. Do you have a few minutes?
Doctor: Not really. I am really backed up. I will not be out of here until 7:00 P.M.
Broker: It's good I caught you then. The sellers are down to $62,500. They need to know by 2:00 P.M. today.
Doctor: It is 1:30 now!
Broker: That's why I am calling. What do you say?

Doctor: Do you think they might take a little less?

Lesson: The physician in this example was ambushed. He was not ready to negotiate, was distracted, and was under so much time pressure that he was not able to practice any good negotiation techniques. In addition, the broker used the veiled threat of an impending deadline to increase the time pressure. This type of call is used repeatedly with physicians. The callers use time limitations to pressure doctors because they know that doctors are frequently too busy to argue. You need to recognize when this technique is being used against you and you need to respond appropriately.

Example 5.5
Broker: Doctor, about the sailboat you and your spouse liked. We are down to crunch time. Do you have a few minutes?
Doctor: No! Give me your number and I will call you back when I am free.
Broker: 508-555-1911. But I need to know....
Doctor: Thank you. Goodbye.

Lesson: In this example, the doctor recognized the ambush and acted appropriately. The doctor will negotiate at the right time—when he is fully prepared and is not distracted. The time pressure has now been effectively shifted to the broker.

You should not commence a negotiation until you are fully prepared. (See pages 27-31 on ambush negotiations.) If someone attempts to begin a negotiation with you at a time when you are not ready, you need to say, "I'm sorry, but I am not ready to discuss this at this time." This policy will keep you from being taken advantage of in an ambush negotiation.

Patience and Pausing

PATIENCE

Physicians are extremely busy people. Many physicians, due to their workloads and hectic schedules, attempt to get the distasteful job of negotiation over as quickly as possible. If your opponent suspects that you fall into this category, you will be at a distinct disadvantage in any negotiation. Consider the following examples.

Example 5.6

Opponent: Thank you, doctor, for joining us. We have several important issues to resolve on your lease and the improvements on the building. We have set aside three hours to work these out. Does that work for you?

Doctor: Three hours? I thought this could be wrapped up in ten minutes. Three hours? Well, I don't know....

Opponent: Well, doctor, we will do the best we can to get you out of here and back to work where you can make some money. Now what kinds of improvements were you looking for?

Lesson: The doctor in this example has placed herself at a distinct disadvantage before formal negotiations have even started. She has revealed that she has not blocked out enough time. Most importantly, the doctor has revealed a lack of patience. This desire to get it over with can be, and usually is, quite costly.

Example 5.7
Opponent: Thank you for joining us. We have several important issues.... How does that work for you?
Doctor: I hope we can wrap it up in three hours. We are committed to getting the improvements we need to run a safe and efficient practice. If we have to discuss this in two or three sessions, so be it. Now, here is a list of the 27 improvements we need. Let's start with number one. The parking situation....

Lesson: The doctor is not rushed and has given a clear, unmistakable message—the negotiation will take as long as necessary.

Patience in negotiations is frequently rewarded with success. Parkinson's Law frequently applies to negotiation sessions: the time taken for decisions is in inverse proportion to the amount of money involved.[2] It makes little sense for you to be too busy to spend the time needed to negotiate over issues involving hundreds of thousands of dollars. The authors recommend "fewer patients but more patience" on the day of an important negotiation.

PAUSING

Successful physician negotiators are able to identify when the key point is reached in a negotiation and when they need some time to think over crucial points, concessions, or decisions. When you reach this point in a negotiation session, **take all the time you need.** There is nothing inherently wrong or embarrassing in saying that you need some time to think something over. Complex negotiation sessions are like a long

---

[2] Recall the shortest physician negotiation on record (pages x-xi).

drive in unfamiliar territory. They contain many forks in the road. You need to make sure that you are on the right road before you proceed. Your opponent will appreciate and respect the fact that you are taking the matter seriously enough to think things over.

If you need a short break you might say that you need to use the rest room or call your partner, spouse, or attorney. This five- to ten-minute break in the negotiation session may be all the time you need to collect yourself and your thoughts and come up with a response or plan. If the matter is more serious and/or you need or want a longer break, you may find that your partner, spouse, or attorney is not readily available. A direct and effective method for continuing the negotiation on another date is to reply, "I need to sleep on that." Any business person understands that this is a good, accepted practice. We have all learned that things frequently look completely different the next day. What was seemingly an insurmountable problem is sometimes resolved easily the next day with a creative solution. What you as a successful physician negotiator want to avoid is the "I wish syndrome," where you wish after a deal is consummated that you had acted differently. Consider the following examples.

Example 5.8
Opponent: Well, doctor, welcome aboard. We have agreed on the salary and fringes. You start next week.
Doctor: Thank you. See you on Monday.
Doctor: (on the way home to himself) I wish I would have remembered to ask for.... If I only said.... I could have gotten....

Lesson: This is the "I wish syndrome." When you sleep on a major negotiation decision, you give yourself time to think things over in a stress-free atmosphere and to reflect on whether you missed anything.

Example 5.9
Opponent: Well, doctor, welcome aboard. We have agreed on the salary and fringes. You start next week.
Doctor: I think we have most of the points covered. I need to review your offer with my spouse and see if we omitted any major items. I will be back at 8:00 A.M. to conclude this and I look forward to starting next week.

Lesson: The doctor has given himself a little wiggle room in case a point was overlooked or omitted in the negotiation session.

You will also need to consider the value of a pause in a concession you may give to an opponent. When you "sleep on it" before you make a concession, the concession will be valued much more than if you assented quickly to a request for the concession. (See pages 139-148 on concessions.) This is another benefit to pausing and sleeping on decisions before deciding key points or making major concessions.

Acceptance Time

All parties in a negotiation session come to the table with their own points of view, ideas, preconceptions, needs, and goals. Negotiation is about obtaining these goals. This can and often does take substantial amounts of time. To get your opponent to change his or her ideas or preconceptions, you will need to allocate adequate time. The successful physician negotiator will anticipate the need for adequate acceptance time and will build it into the negotiation schedule. Consider the following examples.

Example 5.10

Doctor: I am glad we are all here. I decided to cut back on my work schedule. Starting Monday, I will be working half time. Now, let's see if we can work out the finances.

Partners: Phil, we wish you would have given us some lead time, a heads-up or something. I think I speak for all of us when I say we are not ready to talk money. We need more time....

Lesson: The doctor in this case caught his partners by surprise. It was probably not in his best interest to do so. His switching to part time is a radical change that might take his partners time to accept. He may have been better served by allowing them the time needed to be persuaded that things can be worked out satisfactorily for all parties.

Example 5.11

Doctor: (to one partner) Fred, I want to give you a heads-up. In two weeks at the meeting I will be announcing that I will be cutting back to half time. Could you tell the partners? At the meeting, I want to work out scheduling, finances, any loose ends....

Partner: That's quite a surprise. I will let everyone know today. We hate to lose you even half time. But let's see what we can work out.

Lesson: The physician has built some acceptance time into the equation. By the time the negotiation session arrives, the parties are more likely to be cool, collected, and accepting of his decision. They will also be more likely to reach an accommodation that works for all parties.

Deadlines

You must fully understand the use and abuse of deadlines during negotiations. There are nine reasons why deadlines are so important during negotiations. These reasons are listed in Box 5.1. Each reason is discussed in the following subsections.

Box 5.1

Nine Reasons Deadlines Are Important
1. Deadlines make things happen.
2. People respond to and strive to meet deadlines.
3. Deadlines are one of the most powerful and effective tools in the negotiator's arsenal.
4. Deadlines play on the fear of your opponent.
5. Deadlines help reduce your opponent's options.
6. The closer the deadline, the more pressure there is to grant concessions.
7. Objective deadlines can be legitimate and are most effective.
8. Few physicians ask for extensions on deadlines.
9. Accelerated deadlines are effective.

DEADLINES MAKE THINGS HAPPEN

An effective way for a skilled physician negotiator to bring a negotiation to a close is to impose a realistic deadline. If you can get your opponent to buy into the deadline, you have made substantial progress toward closure. Setting a realistic deadline will have the added benefit of reducing the posturing, gamesmanship, brinksmanship, and other tactics that negotiators often employ when they are not facing any deadline. (See pages 177-199 on tactics.)

Example 5.12
Doctor: We agree that we will resolve the remaining issues today and we will stay as long as it takes to do so, agreed?
Opponent: Agreed.

Lesson: The agreement on a deadline by both parties will make it much more likely that an agreement will be reached in a timely fashion.

NEGOTIATORS RESPOND TO AND STRIVE TO MEET DEADLINES

Nobody wants to be known as a person who cannot meet deadlines. Physicians may be particularly sensitive to the need to meet their deadlines because by their nature physicians are achievers. One of the ways you get to be an achiever is by meeting and not questioning deadlines. Your sensitivity to deadlines can be used against you. Consider the following examples.

Example 5.13
Publisher: Your chapter is due June 14 at 5:00 P.M. Eastern Standard Time. It is June 10th. You only have four days left. You know yours is the last chapter we need to send the manuscript to the editor.
Physician: I know…I know…I will have it done. I will work tonight and tomorrow night and have it out to you via an overnight messenger by the 13th. I will not

miss my deadline. I am sorry if I have created any problems.

Lesson: The publisher used the physician's sensitivity to meeting deadlines against the physician. The physician should have considered the actual harm likely to be caused by not meeting the deadline imposed by the publisher.

Example 5.14

Publisher: Your chapter is due June 14th...to send the manuscript to the editor.

Physician: I know. I am running a little behind. I will have it to you in two weeks. This way I will not have to kill myself. In the meantime, why don't you send along the rest of the book to the editor so she can get started and no time is lost?

THE POWER OF DEADLINES

The effective use of deadlines requires you to take a step back and focus not only on your own deadlines, but also on your opponent's deadlines. Once you appreciate the fact that your opponent also has a deadline, you can use that deadline as a powerful negotiating tool. Successful physician negotiators do not obsess unduly about their deadlines.

Example 5.15

Q: You are asked by your partners to lease some office space by March 15, 1998. You are negotiating with an office building owner. It is February 5, 1998, and you are starting to look at the calendar each day. How do deadlines play into this negotiation?

A: How important is your March 15, 1998, deadline? You should talk to your partners and find out whether they really need to move by March 15, 1998. They might give you some more flexibility. The owner says he has no real deadline, but you find out that he is in financial trouble and he needs to rent as soon as possible. You tell him either the deal is completed by February 15, 1998, or you will be forced to go elsewhere. This is an accelerated deadline. If he believes you, he has only ten days to close the negotiation. The more nonchalantly you act, the more nervous he gets. You are using your deadline effectively and can expect increasing concessions from the owner the closer you get to February 15, 1998.

DEADLINES PLAY ON YOUR OPPONENT'S FEARS

The worst fears of your opponent may be that he will fail, not meet his deadline, lose the deal, or will look lazy or incompetent to his employer. By recognizing and playing to these fears, you can use deadlines to your advantage. This can be done quite effectively by phone, e-mail, or fax. Consider the following examples.

Example 5.16
Doctor: (to opponent by phone) If we can't wrap this up by Thursday, I will be looking for another supplier. Thank you.

Lesson: This call puts the deadline "on record" and gives your opponent time to react.

Example 15.17
Doctor: (to opponent by e-mail) Because you have not responded to my calls and letters, I will be closing my file on this matter. Thank you.

Lesson: You as a physician negotiator can use this technique to prod your opponent, raise her anxiety level, and make her respond to your deadlines. This technique has worked well for the authors and in many cases has resulted in the immediate response, "Don't close the file. I was just about to call you...."

Example 15.18
Doctor: (to supervisor of opponent by fax) Please advise if _____ is still employed at your company. I was wondering, as I have been unable to reach her for two weeks. Thank you.

Lesson: This technique can be used to increase the pressure even further on a non-responsive opponent and to play on his *worst* fear, that he may be disciplined by his superior. To comfortably use this technique you need to remember that the goal of negotiation is not to be liked. The goal is to get what you deserve.

DEADLINES HELP REDUCE YOUR OPPONENT'S OPTIONS

Frequently, your opponent will attempt to put off decision making. This is especially true if the decision requires work, commitment, or risk taking. To be successful, you need to simplify an opponent's decisions and make them seem like "no brainers." When your opponent has too many options, decision making and agreement will often be put off.

Example 5.19
Doctor: You have the option of coming on full time, part time, being a consultant, a contractor, or operating on a fee-for-services basis. What do you think?
Opponent: I will have to weigh the pros and cons of each. I will get back to you in a few weeks.

Lesson: The doctor has lost control of this deal. Closing will be delayed while the opponent considers responses to the variety of options offered.

Example 5.20
Doctor: We are offering you half-time work at the salary we discussed. We need to have an answer before the board meeting, which is Tuesday at 10:00 A.M. Remember that sometimes the riskiest course of action is to do nothing.
Opponent: I will get back to you on Monday at the latest.

Lesson: Simplifying the deal, reducing the options, and employing a tight deadline have two benefits. First, you control the direction of the negotiation. Second, you speed up the closing of the deal. These are effective techniques.

THE PRESSURE OF CLOSE DEADLINES

An effective negotiating technique is to find out the time pressures of your opponent and to delay the tough negotiating until a short time before that deadline. This technique uses the accepted negotiation principle that the pressure to grant concessions increases as you get closer to a deadline.[3] (For a full discussion of concessions, see pages 139-148.)

Example 5.21
Physician: (to opponent prospective employee) Your flight leaves in three hours. We have yet to discuss your proposed salary and fringe benefits. I have your demands. As time is short, what is your bottom line? What can you live with? The traffic to the airport will be murder. Maybe you should leave a few minutes early....

Lesson: The doctor is playing off his opponent's time deadline in an attempt to gain concessions.

THE EFFICACY OF OBJECTIVE DEADLINES

An experienced opponent may be somewhat skeptical of your deadlines. She may question whether they are real or just posturing. One way to increase the legitimacy and credibility of your deadline is to make it an "objective" deadline that is difficult or impossible to question. The more concrete, objective, final, and legitimate the deadline, the more likely it is to be taken seriously by your opponent. Some examples of this are provided in Box 5.2.

---

[3] The closer the deadline looms, the *fewer* concessions the skilled physician negotiator will make.

Box 5.2

Objective Deadlines

1. The board is meeting at 3:30 on Tuesday.
2. The lease is up on Friday.
3. I leave for vacation on Wednesday.
4. The flyer will go to the printer at 4:00 P.M.
5. The deal needs to be closed for accounting purposes by Wednesday.
6. We need to resolve this before the weather turns bad.
7. We have other bids we need to respond to by 3:30.
8. Our fiscal year ends on June 30.
9. I am currently in negotiations with your competitors. If we don't have your proposal by tomorrow, we're going with the competition.
10. For tax reasons, this needs to be done by December 31.

THE EXTENSION OF DEADLINES

Few physician negotiators ask for extensions. They should. By failing to do so they effectively accept their opponent's deadlines and become trapped by their parameters. Opponents will use your preoccupation with the deadline against you. Do not let them. In the rare cases in which the deadline cannot be extended, figure out what will happen if you miss the deadline. You should then perform a quick mental cost-benefit analysis. You need to determine whether meeting the deadline is as important as obtaining your goals. Frequently it is not. Consider the following examples.

Example 5.22
Opponent: Well, doctor, I know you have a few additional items you would like, but we have only 45 minutes left. Why don't you cut down your wish list to its bare essentials and let's see what we can do?

Lesson: You will not lose face or damage your reputation by requesting an extension of a deadline. When you need or want an extension of a deadline, you should ask for it as soon as you suspect you need it. You should also make sure the extension is long enough.

Example 5.23
Doctor: (to opponent) We have four or five more items to cover. I am committed to trying to resolve these issues and reach an agreement. I am willing to stay two hours beyond the 3:00 P.M. deadline. Does that work for you?

Lesson: The doctor put subtle pressure on the opponent by questioning her commitment to reaching an agreement. She did *not* accept her deadline as inviolate.

When the stakes are high and the negotiators committed, no deadline, no matter how firm or absolute, cannot be changed, modified, or worked around.

Example 5.24
During the 1998 peace negotiations in Northern Ireland, after years of negotiations, the parties were running up

against their absolute "drop-dead" deadline. They were so close to an agreement that facilitator Senator George Mitchell and the other parties agreed to "unplug" the clock to give themselves the extra 24 hours they needed to reach the Good Friday Agreement.

Lesson: Almost all deadlines can be extended.

THE IMPORTANCE OF ACCELERATED DEADLINES

An accelerated deadline occurs when you tell your opponent that you need the issue resolved prior to when it actually needs to be resolved. Accelerated deadlines are important because your opponent will normally wait until the last possible moment to act. If you do not give yourself an adequate buffer of time, you might not have enough time to explore and close alternative deals.

Example 5.25
Q: A doctor needed an organization to give him some documents he required for tax purposes. He needed them to claim a charitable donation of royalties. There was an intense negotiation going on. Finally, in September 1997, the doctor gave them a deadline: "Either I have the documents from you by December 31, 1997, or the deal is off." What is wrong with the deadline employed in the above example?
A: The doctor failed to give an accelerated deadline to build in time for problems that could be reasonably anticipated. The doctor should have given a much shorter deadline. The deadline permits negotiations until midnight December 31, 1997, and it allows no time for mistakes, snowstorms, acts of God, clerical errors, or review by counsel. This doctor will be helpless if his opponents fax him a letter on December 31, 1997, at 4:00 P.M. He has boxed himself in

unnecessarily. An accelerated deadline of November 24, 1997, would have been more appropriate.

<u>Conclusion</u>

The successful physician negotiator needs to understand the proper use of deadlines. He will research his opponent's deadlines, set his opponent's deadlines as short as possible, not obsess about his own deadlines, request an extension when necessary, and use accelerated deadlines liberally.

Chapter 6 How to Gain Power in a Negotiation

To be successful, you need to identify the sources of power in your negotiations and use these sources effectively. *Power* in negotiating means the ability to exercise authority and influence. The ability or perceived ability to get things done is also power. The sources of power or perceived power by physician negotiators are numerous and are limited only by the negotiator's creativity and imagination. If you can convince your opponent that you are in control, you will have gained power.

Knowledge Is Power

Preparation and information will greatly increase your power. (See pages 117-132 on preparation.) You will be at a distinct advantage if you have done your homework. You should have at your fingertips all of the pertinent statistical, financial, and historical data. You will also need to know about your opponent's needs, desires, and pressures, as well as her business organization and its structure. The most important knowledge for you to obtain is the real, as opposed to the expressed, needs of your opponent. This knowledge can rapidly shift the balance of power in your favor.

Finding out information requires research. As part of this research, you may want to consider talking to physicians who have already gone through similar negotiations. You will also need to ask a lot of questions. Timid, shy, and unquestioning doctors will not be good negotiators. Knowledge is power. Obtain it and use it to your advantage.

Example 6.1
Opponent: We know you would like to sell your practice and we can offer you one-and-a-half times gross in stock in our company with a one-year employment agreement. We will need a five-year covenant not to compete in this state.
Doctor: As a publicly traded company your financial and acquisition history is a matter of public record. We have checked your SEC form 10Q and your annual report. After reviewing these documents and talking to the heads of the last five practices you acquired, we know that you have paid up to 2.5 times gross with 50% cash and 50% stock. The one-year employment contract is considerably shorter than the one you offered x, y, and z, and the covenant not to compete is twice as long as Dr. Hardball signed. In addition, we are concerned about the way you treated Drs. Smith and Cohen after their acquisition.

Lesson: This is a doctor who has done her homework. She has thoroughly researched her opponent and is therefore in a strong position to obtain more favorable terms.

Example 6.2
Background: A physician we know was negotiating to sell his practice to a multi-state group. The negotiations were stalled until he found out that this new company was planning to go public shortly and needed to quickly acquire the licenses his practice maintained. After some tough negotiating, he obtained an excellent offer for his practice of six times his gross revenue.

Lesson: Knowledge is power. By determining that the opponent needed to purchase his practice, the physician was able to obtain very favorable terms.

Alternatives

You should *always* walk into negotiations with several options. You can then compare these options to your opponent's proposal, use them as a benchmark, and, when helpful, show them to your opponent to obtain a better deal. You also need to be aware of the possible options of your opponent. You gain power in negotiations when you have more alternatives at your disposal than your opponent does. You are at a tremendous disadvantage when you have no other alternatives and absolutely need to make a deal with your opponent.

Example 6.3

Doctor: As you know, we would like to book our medical convention for 1999. We need 400 sleeping rooms, meeting rooms for 800 (classroom style), and we will have continental breakfasts and lunches and maybe another food and beverage function.

Hotel sales manager: We can accommodate you. We need you to sign a $100,000 cancellation clause and an attrition clause indicating that your organization will agree to pay for all the rooms not rented. Here is our standard form....

Doctor: We know about the medical conventions you lost last year and the trouble you had. We do not sign $100,000 cancellation clauses and do not sign any attrition clauses. Here are two proposed contracts from four-star hotels in this area. If you meet their terms we can talk. If not.... By the way, this will be an annual event. We will be making a decision in 48 hours.

Lesson: A combination of techniques was used successfully to attempt to negotiate a better contract. They include knowledge of lost meetings, research on the opponent, developing options, having information readily available, and knowing exactly what the options were. It is hard for an opponent to argue against a written contract proposal from a competitor. You need to define your options clearly so that they can be used at the negotiation session.

Industry Standards

It may be useful to demonstrate that your proposal or terms are the industry standard or accepted practice. You can use this fact to gain power in the negotiation. The result can be that your opponent is no longer negotiating against you, but instead against the industry. It is best to bring in the documents, facts, and figures and to have them available to lay on the table. If your opponent was unaware of the industry standards or unaware that you were aware of them, your power will be increased.

Example 6.4
Doctor: I would love to write and edit a national newsletter for you on medical ethics. I understand it will be published bimonthly. How about $4,500 an issue?
Publisher: With your national reputation the newsletter will be great! Doctor, we publish twelve other medical newsletters. We pay a straight 10% royalty payable annually. Here are the contracts for the

other newsletters. The 10% is standard in the industry. Feel free to check around. If you are not interested....
Doctor: The 10% will be fine. When do I start?

Lesson: The publisher's knowledge of industry standards increased her power.

Expertise

It may be useful to portray yourself as an expert. If you do, your opponent could have a tendency to treat you respectfully and to defer to your expertise. To appear to be an expert, you need to give the perception that you have superior knowledge, expertise, experience, information, or technical skills. Note that if you need to obtain information directly from your opponent, making yourself out as an expert could make this more difficult. (See pages 49-51 on playing dumb.) Also note that when this technique is used against you, you should cite your own experts and refuse to buy or sign anything you don't understand. Consider the following examples.

Example 6.5
Doctor: As I understand this proposal, you would like us to set up a telemedicine service for your multinational company to increase quality of service and hold down costs. Is that correct?
Entrepreneur: Yes. In essence, that's it.
Doctor: I assume the reason you are here is because we have written the text on telemedicine and have developed the standard in interactive computer services.
Entrepreneur: Yes. You are the experts.
Doctor: To make this happen and run a high quality service, we will need the following computer

equipment...; the following staff...; and a budget annually of.... In the long run, you will increase the quality of medical care and hold down costs.

Lesson: The doctor/expert has used her superior, acknowledged technical expertise and experience as powerful negotiating tools.

Example 6.6

Salesperson: As you know, doctor, we developed the fax on demand system. What your practice needs is the supercharged 179 system that costs $29,400. Should we draw up the contract?

Doctor: We have retained Ms. Hartley as a consultant. I am sure you have heard of her. She recommends the 119 system and told us not to spend more than $14,500. Before we even get to which model to consider, I have a simple rule of life. I do not purchase or invest in anything I do not fully understand. Can you break this down so someone without a Ph.D. in computer science can understand it? I have set aside ten minutes for this meeting.

Lesson: By employing her own expert/consultant, refusing to sign anything that is not understood, and setting a tight deadline, the physician in the above example has neutralized the expertise of the salesperson and regained the power and control over the negotiation.

Investment

The more effort, expense, time, and emotional energy your opponent has invested in the negotiation, the more your power has increased. Such an investment of time and effort is an indication of your opponent's strong desire to close a deal. After hours, days, or weeks of ongoing negotiation, your opponent does not want to go back to his boss and tell her that he could not reach an agreement. Psychologically, once your opponent has sensed, decided, or in the best case, informed his superior that a deal is close, it is very difficult for that person to walk away. In such a case he has invested psychic energy and can almost taste the agreement. Anything less is seen as a personal and professional failure. You need to recognize the power of investment and use it to your advantage when negotiating.

Example 6.7
Doctor: This is your third and, as far as I am concerned, your final sales call. The $72,000 system you are trying to sell us is priced too high. I know you put a lot of time and money into your presentations and demonstrations. I am sorry. I have to run.
Computer salesperson: (sensing a sale slipping away) I hate to see this fall through over a few dollars. What if we reduced the price 5%?
Doctor: Maybe we can reconsider this next year. Thanks again.
Salesperson: (a little more desperate) What will it take to make this sale?
Doctor: A 10% price reduction, two years free service, and the software we discussed. We would need installation within one week.
Salesperson: Give me five minutes to call my sales manager.

Lesson: The physician used the fact that the salesperson was more invested in the deal than she was to her advantage.

Legitimacy and Precedents

You should use precedents and/or legitimacy to increase your power during negotiations. For example, people generally do not question hotel check-in policies of 2:00 P.M. and checkout policies of 11:00 A.M. This is a result of the power of precedents and legitimacy. This policy is printed on the official notices on the inside of the hotel doors and is the way "everyone" does it.

When you receive a standard form, set price, usual and customary mark up, 16% service charge, or penalty for early withdrawal, you see the power of legitimacy and precedents in action against you. This type of power is unquestioned and self-perpetuating. If the reason you pay X is because it has always been X and everyone else is paying X, you and everyone else will always pay X. You need to be able to use this technique to your own advantage. You also need to be able to effectively respond to it when it's used against you. The best way to do this is to make your situation appear to be unique, thus meriting special consideration.

Example 6.8

Corporate sponsor: We would like to be a corporate sponsor for your upcoming medical meeting.
Doctor: Fine. That will be $25,000 and we will need you to pay for the lunch as well.
Corporate sponsor: Well, we didn't really plan on spending that much.
Doctor: The $25,000 fee is set by the Board. Here is the resolution. It has been unchanged for three years. As a matter of fact, it is less than the sponsorship requirements of these three comparable medical

seminars (handing him documents). We do have another party interested.

Corporate sponsor: Let me make a few calls. I will get back to you this afternoon.

Lesson: The physician effectively used precedents, legitimacy, knowledge, alternatives, industry standards, and time pressure. As in many cases when this power technique is used effectively, the discussion never turns to whether $25,000 plus the food and beverages was a fair price because it was *the* price.

Example 6.9

Doctor: Our rate for capitation compensation is $600 per patient.

Opponent: I'm sorry, doctor, the set price in our standard contract is $500 per patient.

Doctor: Our standard rate is $600 per patient. We are currently receiving that from companies X, Y, and Z. We are the most prestigious practice in this part of the state. Without us, you'll never have a strong following here.

Opponent: I appreciate that, doctor, but $500 is our standard rate.

Doctor: Standard service rates a standard rate. Our practice delivers exceptionally good care. Have you had a chance to read the 100 letters of recommendation from our patients that I sent to you? If your doctors give standard care in this industry you'll never get anyone to sign up for your plan. Our practice is proven to be of the highest quality and as such our rate is $600 per patient.

Opponent: You may have a point. Let me talk to my boss and get back to you later.

Lesson: The physician successfully set his practice apart from others that were receiving the standard rate. He employed other precedents and used his own standard rate, which he justified, as a way to gain movement on his opponent's set price.

Example 6.10
Background: A doctor and his wife go away off-season to a beach resort community to have a romantic Saturday night. They prefer to stay at Inn X. Inn X's large parking lot is empty when they arrive.

Doctor: I'd like to get a room for the night please. What's your rate?
Innkeeper: Our standard rates are published on this card...$119 per night.
Doctor: Wow, that's pretty steep for January. I was quoted $69 per night at Inn Y and that place has a Jacuzzi. Listen, this place is nearly empty. We'd love to stay here and give you the business, but we need to get a rate of $69 per night.
Innkeeper: Fine. We'd love to have you. Let's do it for $69. I'll need to see a major credit card.

Lesson: *Everything* is negotiable. This is especially true of standard rates or prices.

Coping with Uncertainty

You need to be able to cope with uncertainty and react appropriately to unforeseen events. Such flexibility increases your negotiation power. If you follow a script or plan strictly, no matter how well thought out and well prepared, you will be at a distinct disadvantage and will decrease your negotiation power. This is true because your inflexibility will be perceived as a sign of weakness and a lack of expertise and sophistication. If your opponent senses your inflexibility, he may start to throw you curve balls, red herrings, or negotiation bombshells to see how you react.

Example 6.11
Real estate agent: We can rent this space to you for $4,500 a month.
Doctor: We need to get a long-term lease, medical upgrading so we don't get invoiced, buildout costs, and the right to sublet or assign.
Real estate agent: We can work with those requirements as long as we get a triple net lease.
Doctor: We have never signed anything like that before. It will not be acceptable.

Lesson: The doctor has potentially lost a very good deal. He obtained all the terms he was seeking. However, his inflexibility in not even considering the triple net lease has worked strongly to his disadvantage. The doctor needed to be more flexible and to prepare for the unexpected.

Persistence

Persistence pays off. Physicians who are relentless, who do not back down or give up, and who continue to come back to their central points increase their power in negotiations. Once you are able to convince your opponents that you will not give in, they start to think, "What is it going to take to get this person to sign off?"
Successful physician negotiators are not worn down and do not give up on their central points because a negotiation is taking too long. They know a

negotiation will take as long as necessary. When you feel you are right and project the sincerity of your belief to your opponent, you start to raise his or her anxiety level and increase your power in the negotiation process.[1]

Example 6.12

Attorney: Doctor, we have been over this three or four times already. We cannot get you the $189,000. Be reasonable. Compromise and let's be done with it. We are both losing more time and money than this is worth.
Doctor: I don't care if we go over this 44 times. I do *not* back down when I am right. And I am right. You know it and I know it. I will continue to stick to the price unless I am convinced otherwise. As to wasting time and money, unfortunately I cannot bill $250 an hour like you do.

Lesson: Persistence can give you power and it often pays off.

Example 6.13

Attorneys are professional negotiators. The top negotiator at one of Boston's largest law firms has been described to the authors as the best for one overriding reason: his relentless persistence. He has been described as follows, "Absolutely relentless, will not move on and come back to a difficult point later. Always has another persuasive argument ready to go."

---

[1] Remember, "persistence is to power, what carbon is to steel." Cohen, 83.

Sole Source

In nearly every physician's life there will be one or more golden business opportunities when he or she is the only game in town. You may have expertise, knowledge, programs, or products that are not available elsewhere or at least are perceived as difficult, if not impossible, to replace. The successful physician negotiator will actively pursue putting herself into this position and will capitalize on this when it occurs. When you are the sole source of information, products, programs, and expertise, many of the standard negotiation rules do not apply. You should no longer concern yourself with or be bound by industry standards, legitimacy, and precedent. The truth is quite simple. Number one, you have what they want. Number two, you are worth whatever they are willing to pay and whatever you are willing accept. Nothing else matters!

Example 6.14

Attorney: As the leading expert on the AMA *Guides*, we want you to fly down to Texas to testify on the issue of its fairness and constitutionality.
Doctor: No, I am too busy.
Attorney: We will pay you $200 an hour.
Doctor: I am too busy.
Attorney: We will pay you $300 an hour.
Doctor: I am too busy.
Attorney: Okay. What will it take?
Doctor: $350 an hour portal to portal, airfare, and out-of-pocket expenses with a $15,000 retainer.
Attorney: But the testimony with travel will be three days...72 hours at $350 an hour.
Doctor: Exactly.

Attorney: Okay.[2]

Lesson: The doctor was uniquely qualified. He was the sole source. As such, he was able to command extremely favorable terms. All that was required was that he ask and hold out for them.

Conclusion

Acting as if you do have power will increase your opponent's perception of your power in any negotiation. Emphasize and demonstrate your knowledge and expertise. Develop your options and alternatives. Use industry standards, the power of investment, legitimacy, persistence, and flexibility to your advantage. Position yourself whenever possible to become the sole source. If you can, don't be afraid to capitalize on it. Perception *is* reality in negotiation. When you act as if you have power, your opponent will perceive that you actually have power. When your opponent perceives your power, you will be able to negotiate better deals.

---

[2] This example is based upon an actual event.

Chapter 7 Preparing to Win

Proper preparation is essential. Thorough and well thought-out preparation increases the likelihood of success. Preparation requires you to properly execute a negotiation plan. This plan should identify the issues, your goals, and the likely goals of your opponent. The three preparatory stages are:

1. information gathering,
2. analysis, and
3. planning.

Recognize When You Are Negotiating

The single biggest mistake physicians make is not adequately preparing for negotiation. The reasons that physicians frequently do not properly prepare for negotiations are not dissimilar from why they often do not bother to negotiate at all. (See pages 7-9 on why physicians don't negotiate.) In many cases, the unsuccessful physician negotiator is not prepared because he does not even recognize that he is involved in a negotiation. The physician negotiator who fails to identify when he is, or should be, negotiating cannot prepare for the negotiation. (See pages 27-31 where we discuss ambush negotiation.) Consider the following examples.

Example 7.1
Media advance person: Doctor, we would like to interview you for an hour for our cable show on informed consent on June 1, 1999. For your

convenience, we will come to your office at 1:00 P.M.
Okay?
Doctor: Fine. Should I wear a blue shirt and a solid
tie?

Lesson: The physician never bothered to prepare
because he failed to identify that he was involved in a
negotiation.

Example 7.2
Media advance person: Doctor, we would like to
interview you.... Okay?
Doctor: This sounds interesting, but I am quite busy.
Please fax me the names and phone numbers of the last
four doctors you interviewed, as I will need to talk to
them. I will need you to include in the fax how long
this taping will take, what preparation I will need to do,
what you intend to do with the interview, and what my
compensation will be for my participation. I will call
you this week to see if we can reach an agreement.

Lesson: The doctor identified the negotiation
opportunity and bought some time to investigate and
properly prepare for the negotiation session ahead.
This doctor can then call the other doctors who were
interviewed and see how they were compensated, if the
advance person's time predictions were accurate, and if
the interview was a pleasant experience.

Physicians Are Too Busy to Prepare

Many physicians do not bother to prepare for
negotiations because they do not have the time to do so.
These physicians are too busy seeing patients, filling
out paperwork, dealing with office staff, etc. The

resulting lack of preparation puts these physicians at a
distinct disadvantage in the negotiation. It is a chief
reason for their poor results. In any significant
negotiation, the time you spend preparing will *save,* not
cost, you money. If you do not have the time to devote
to the preparation, get some help or have someone else
negotiate for you.

Example 7.3
Q: You are about to negotiate to buy a new Volvo.
You know where the information is available on the
Internet regarding what the dealer pays for them, but
don't have time to play with the computer for an hour
and then crunch all the numbers. What should you do?
A: Delay your visit to the showroom until you do have
the time to do the research. Alternatively, assign
someone else, say a teenage child, to do the research for
you and present it to you in an easy-to-understand
format.

How to Prepare

Recognizing the need for preparation and setting aside
the time for it are only the first steps. You next need to
know *how* to prepare. You should first identify the
issues to be negotiated and then set your goals and
anticipate the likely objectives of the opponent.

ISSUES

You will need to fully and completely identify the
issues. This task should be accomplished promptly.
Doing so in a timely fashion will leave you adequate
time for further preparation. As the following example
shows, it can often be advantageous if you position

yourself, as opposed to your opponent, to define the issues to be discussed.

Example 7.4
Doctor: Jim, I am faxing you the agenda for our meeting next week. As I understand it, the issues are annual salary, medical and dental benefits, vacation, hours, and coverage. Did I miss anything?
Prospective employee: No, that covers it. Fax it along. Thank you.

Lesson: The physician negotiator seized control of the negotiation by preparing the agenda. The order of issues and time allocations in the agenda can be important in maintaining control over the negotiation session. If they are ever reached, issues placed at the end of the agenda with short time allocations will be discussed only briefly.

GOALS

Successful physician negotiators recognize that they need to set realistically high goals. It is a well-accepted negotiation axiom that negotiators who start with high aspiration levels (but not so high as to be unrealistic) achieve better results than those who aim lower. High aspiration levels that are logical, dependable, and make sense are often extremely effective in a negotiation. Unsuccessful physician negotiators may set their goals too low because they are afraid to lose and afraid to fail.

Before you can achieve your goals, you need to set them. Once you have laid out your goals and the likely objectives of your opponent, you can begin information gathering in earnest.

In setting goals, it is best to identify what you are trying to achieve, the least you can offer (and still be realistic), the most you can offer (and still be satisfied with the result), and your best alternative. It also is very important for you to put yourself in the shoes of your opponent and attempt to anticipate what she sees as her goals, lowest offer, best offer, and alternative.

You will be more convincing if you honestly believe that your position is reasonable. In other words, first convince yourself. It will then be easier to convince your opponent. You should use research, information, objective data and statistics, and precedents to help convince yourself about the correctness of your position.

Example 7.5

Background: A physician is preparing to negotiate for the purchase of a group medical practice. She makes the following plan:

Goal	To acquire successful specialty practice in geographic proximity to current practice to increase income and compliment practice.
Least can offer	One times their gross annual receipts
Most can offer	Two-and-a-half times their gross annual receipts
Best alternative	Acquire similar practice 30 miles away. (Tentative offer to sell at one-and-a-half times gross revenue.)
Other	They need to sell more than we need to buy.

Anticipated opponent's position

Goal	To sell their practice. (The doctors want to retire.)
Most will demand	Four times gross
Least will accept	One times gross
Best alternative	To find another purchaser in same area with same specialty focus. (Difficult to locate.)
Other	Desperate to sell.

Lesson: The seller has thoroughly prepared. By putting all the important information in front of her, she can rationally determine how much she should offer and how she should respond to the demands of the seller.

Information Gathering

The five W's of journalism are when, who, what, where, and why. These five W's are a good guide to the type of information you should gather prior to a negotiating session.

WHEN

Start to gather information as early as possible.[1] This should begin well before the formal negotiation session starts. The closer you get to the negotiation session, the harder it is to obtain information. You also need to leave yourself a little extra time in case the information

---

[1] "How do you gather information? You start early, because the earlier you start, the easier it is to obtain information. You can always get more information preceding an acknowledged, formal confrontation, because people willingly let their hair down...once...their attitude becomes defensive, they say, 'Come on...I can't tell you anything now. It's negotiation time.'" Cohen, 102.

you sought turns out to be harder to gather than you anticipated.

Example 7.6

Q: You have scheduled a negotiation session to discuss employment with a large health insurer. You realize that you should review the company's SEC filings published on the Internet prior to the negotiation. One hour before the meeting you go on-line to get the company's latest annual report and proxy statements. Unfortunately, the server is down and the information cannot be retrieved. What have you done wrong?

A: By waiting until the last minute to gather information, you will not be able to respond to the contingency of the server being down. If you had tried to obtain the information one week ahead of time, there would have been ample time remaining to secure it.

WHO

Talk to anyone who can help you gather information. Do not be shy. Do not be an elitist. Start from the bottom up. Talk to clerks, janitors, secretaries, assistants, patients, colleagues, former partners, business associates, spouses, and former spouses. Do not ask inappropriate questions and try, where appropriate, to maintain anonymity. Be aware that some of your questions may find their way back to your opponent. It is often appropriate to ask for an information package directly from the person you will be negotiating with. Don't be afraid to ask for any and all information. You will often be pleasantly surprised at what you will get.

Example 7.7

You are negotiating an employment agreement for yourself at a group practice. You want to know how busy the practice is. You call up and tell the receptionist that you are a new patient and would like to get an appointment. She informs you that it will take five weeks.

Lesson: By going to the receptionist for information, you have learned that the group is very busy. This is important because it means that they may be desperate to make a hire. It is also important because you may suspect that you may be overworked if you take the job.

WHAT

Seek out any type of information that can help you to prepare. For example, if you are dealing with public companies, seek out on the Internet, or elsewhere, their public filings, annual reports, SEC filings, etc. The company itself will, if requested, send you a catalog, advertisements, and press releases. Getting on their mailing list can be very beneficial. Searches on the Internet can provide a wealth of information, ranging from your opponent's CV to the company's business plan.

Example 7.8

A small, publicly held corporation is negotiating with you for the acquisition of your practice. They have offered you 20,000 shares of their company's stock. You research the company's stock performance record through the Internet. You learn that five years ago their stock was trading at 90, that it fell to a low of 2, and it is now up to 6. They state that the stock is "going places."

Lesson: Your research indicates a shaky performance for the company's stock. You should strongly consider insisting upon cash.

WHERE

There are few limits on where you can seek out information to prepare for your negotiation. As a successful physician negotiator, you or a member of your staff can use specialized business or medical libraries, on-line services, inside reports, or articles written by or papers delivered by your opponent. The depth of your information gathering should depend upon the amount at stake in the negotiation. When lawyers prepare for a significant case, they frequently obtain and read everything their opponent and/or experts have ever written or delivered orally. In negotiations that include substantial amounts, the successful physician negotiator should do no less.

Example 7.9
You are considering selling your practice to a company headed by "Chainsaw" Al Smith. You would like to stay on at the practice for five more years, then retire. You perform a literature search on Mr. Smith. You learn from old *Wall Street Journal* articles that he is called "Chainsaw" Al because he has a reputation of taking over businesses and firing most of its high level employees.

Lesson: After conducting this research you may want to consider demanding an airtight five-year employment contract. You might also want to consider finding a job somewhere else or not selling to this buyer.

WHY

The more you know about what motivates your opponent, the more likely you are to achieve your goals in the negotiation. (See pages 76-82 on what makes your opponent tick.)

Example 7.10
You are negotiating a business deal with the CEO of a mid-sized company. One day, when talking with his secretary, you discover that he is an avid golfer. You send him a case of highly prized golf balls from "one straight shooter to another."

Lesson: This act of good will, based on information regarding the opponent's passion for golf, can only help to facilitate the upcoming negotiations.

Analysis

A careful analysis must be made once all the information is gathered. You need to analyze the facts and arguments and then challenge the underlying assumptions upon which they are based. You should not assume to know what the other party wants, desires, or thinks is important in a negotiation. Physicians frequently assume that:

> 1. their opponent will act as they would if they were in the same situation,
> 2. their opponent will act logically, and
> 3. their opponent will do what is in his or her best interest.

Each of these basic assumptions is flawed.

ASSUMPTION #1: YOUR OPPONENT WILL ACT AS YOU WOULD

Do not assume that your opponent will act as you do. If you do, you will essentially be looking in the mirror and negotiating with yourself. Making this assumption can lead to poor results.

Example 7.11
Doctor: We appreciate all your hard work and will "take care of you" during bonus time.
Colleague: I appreciate it, but that doesn't solve my problem. The traveling I am doing is wreaking havoc with my spouse and kids. I am never around on weekends. I missed the last three soccer matches,...I was the only parent that wasn't there during the annual show at school. Instead I was stuck at an airport hotel. I am very close to leaving.

Lesson: The doctor is wrong in assuming that money, in the form of a bonus, will resolve the problem. This could be a very costly assumption. What his colleague may really be concerned with is the time away from his family. A bonus will not fix this problem. The doctor needed to employ better active listening skills. (See pages 64-82 on active listening techniques and pages 68-69 on hearing what is *not* being said.)

ASSUMPTION #2: YOUR OPPONENT WILL ACT LOGICALLY

Frequently, physician negotiators assume they know what their opponent will do because it is the logical thing to do. This assumption is dangerous. *People do not always do what is logical.* (See pages 161-168 on emotions.) You also need to consider that when your opponent is under pressures or stresses that you are unaware of, actions that would seem illogical to you may seem very logical to your opponent.

Example 7.12
Doctor: Phil, are you telling me that you are going to give up the practice of medicine, move to Cape Cod, and open a few bagel shops?
Partner: That's right—less hassles, more family time, less pressures....
Doctor: Phil, that's crazy. Your lost income, the goodwill, the patients....
Partner: I am forty-nine. It is now or never. I will be having some fun.

Lesson: What seems illogical to you may seem very logical to someone with different values. Just because your opponents are doing something that appears to be illogical, it doesn't mean that they are being illogical in their own minds. Again, you need to find out what makes your opponent tick.

ASSUMPTION #3: YOUR OPPONENT WILL DO WHAT IS IN HIS OR HER BEST INTEREST

Even when it is clear to you what is in the best interest of your opponent, he may still not take that course of action. This fact is difficult for physician negotiators to accept. It occurs because often your opponent assumes different things than you would assume if you were in her position. It also occurs because some people simply make flawed decisions.

Example 7.13
The authors had a set of medical videos placed
exclusively in a catalog. The videos were selling well.
At the end of the exclusivity period, we informed the
catalog owner that we would start to market the videos
ourselves to a completely different market. The catalog
company owner could continue to sell the videos in his
catalog at the same terms. The catalog owner was
insulted in our lack of confidence in his catalog and no
amount of logical argument or proof would change his
mind. He dropped the set of videos. This was truly a
lose/lose conclusion, because both parties lost money
for no logical reason. It seemed to us that it was clearly
in his best interest to continue to sell the videos. That is
the reason why we did not renew the exclusive
arrangement.

Planning

Once you have set your goals, anticipated the likely
objectives of your opponent, and gathered all the
information available and analyzed it, you are ready to
move to the final preparation stage. This stage involves
the preparation of a negotiation plan. The successful
physician negotiator carefully plans each aspect of the
negotiation session from the location (see pages 33-37)
to the tactics to be used (see pages 177-199). You need
to think of yourself not only as the actor, but as the
producer, director, choreographer, and stage director as
well. Your negotiation plan needs to be well thought
out. The authors use the decision tree model as an
effective negotiation planning device.

As former trial lawyers, we always prepare our
case *and* the other side's case. We put ourselves in the
other lawyer's shoes. What will she argue? How
should we respond? What are our weak points? There

are four elements we concentrate on. These elements are listed in Box 7.1.

Box 7.1

Preparation Points

1. What is the opponent's *position* likely to be?
2. What is the opponent's *rationale* likely to be?
3. What are the opponent's *weak and strong points*?
4. Where is the opponent most *vulnerable*—(on the opening position, the fall back, or the bottom line)?

The use of a decision tree can be very helpful in avoiding surprises. It allows you to prepare to react "spontaneously" to events in the negotiation. In reality, however, you have had time to think through in advance the logical consequences of your response. Successful physician negotiators who effectively employ their decision trees are like chess grand masters. Like grand masters, they are prepared for every move of the opponent and have played the game out several times in advance before their next move.

Example 7.14
A decision tree for a simple negotiation follows.

Employment negotiation
Salary
If they offer less than $150,00 a year: sticking point (must meet this base salary or else catch early flight back).

If they meet or exceed $150,00 a year: move to health and dental insurance.

Insurance
Malpractice: Mandatory: nonnegotiable
Health Insurance: Mandatory: nonnegotiable; full
                      family coverage
Dental Insurance: Negotiable: (get if can)

Length of contract
Ideal: 2 years (for flexibility)
Lowest: 1 year (security)
Highest: 3 years (do not want to be
                      boxed in)

[NOTE: If they demand more than three years, revisit
salary and ask for cost of living increases: A) based on
rate of inflation and B) other standard.]

On-call status
Ideal: 1 day per month
Highest: 3 days per month

[NOTE: If 2 days or more, ask for compensatory pay to
discourage additional coverage time. Propose sliding
scale downward with passage of time for on-call dates.]

Vacation
Ideal: 5 weeks per year
Minimum: 3 weeks per year

[NOTE: Fight hard: "rationale"—need to stay fresh and
not "burn-out." Tie into length of contract if less than 4
weeks, no more than 2-year contract.]

Perks
Moving expenses: Ask for $4,500; take $2,500
Sick days: Ask for 10; take 5; if need be,
                      talk "team player"

Income from other sources: Ask to keep 100% (can
                             cap at $20,000 if need to).
Noncompetition clause: "Talk trust" and give
                             away as little as possible.
                             Have attorney check.
                             Blame her if need be.

Lesson: The decision tree forces the physician
negotiator to prepare and anticipate problems. Once
prepared, the physician has persuasive arguments and
rationales readily available. The decision tree also
enables the negotiator to see the big picture and to
demonstrate how all the terms in an agreement are
interdependent.

Chapter 8 Silence Is Golden

You will need to be able to keep silent when necessary. Silence is a potent strategic weapon. It can also be an excellent method of communicating. It can, however, often be one of the most difficult communication skills for physicians to master.

Strategic Weapon

You should let your opponent talk first and let her do most of the talking. This requires self-discipline.[1] If you are able to listen more than you talk, you will accomplish a chief aim of the negotiation because you will get more information than you give. (See pages 39-82 and 122-126 on gathering information.) Just as nature abhors a vacuum, a weak negotiator abhors silence. You need to realize that silence may make your opponent very uncomfortable. The longer the silence goes on, the more excruciating it can be for your opponent. Your opponent will frequently talk to fill the void and keep the negotiation going. The more your opponent talks to fill the void, the more likely she will be to inadvertently disclose information you can use or to make a key concession. Consider the following examples.

Example 8.1
Seller: We are asking $395,000 for the office building.
Doctor: (long silence)

---

[1] Above all, you need to avoid the temptation to prove how smart you are by continuously talking.

Seller: We do have some flexibility. How much are you looking to pay?

Lesson: Silence can immediately raise the anxiety level of your opponent. He could be thinking to himself, "Am I too high? Am I off base? Have I angered my opponent?" The doctor's silence resulted directly in the concession of flexibility on the issue of price.

Example 8.2
Consider the movie *The Caine Mutiny*. In the film, José Ferrer cross-examines the Captain (Humphrey Bogart) in order to try and prove that he was mentally unstable and unfit for command. He questions the Captain until he goes off on a long and disjointed verbal tirade on the missing strawberries and other topics. At the end of the tirade, the Captain proved through his own conduct that he was unfit for command. This gambit worked only because José Ferrer's character was disciplined and sophisticated enough to keep silent and let his opponent hang himself.

Silence is also an effective way of increasing the significance given to what you eventually do say. When you do not speak often, your words take on heightened significance. Consider the following example.

Example 8.3
At a recent negotiation session, there were eight doctors, three insurance representatives, and one attorney in attendance. All of the physicians and others

at the meeting fully expressed themselves about the matter at issue. For forty-five minutes the attorney sat silent. At the end of forty-five minutes, one of the doctors said, "We have not heard from Steve. Steve, what do you have to say?" The room quieted and the attorney's comments were singled out. They were treated with more attention and respect than they probably deserved. Silence was used to amplify what was eventually said in the negotiation session.

Method of Communication

Remaining silent after your opponent has made an offer or proposal can be effective. This technique may quickly reduce your opponent's aspiration levels. In addition, remaining silent gives you the added protection of not making any verbal leaks of information. Consider the following examples.

Example 8.4

Insurer: Doctor, your outstanding medical bill is $3,892.00. As you know, we are disputing coverage and the services rendered. We will offer you $2,000 to settle this bill today.
Doctor: (silence)

Lesson: Although the doctor has said nothing, he has quickly and decisively communicated his displeasure with the offer made. In addition, it is much harder for his opponent to read the doctor. There are no verbal cues or leaks. (See page 70 on verbal leaks.)

Example 8.5
Insurer: Doctor, your outstanding bill is $3,892.00.
We will offer $2,000 to settle this bill today.
Doctor: I think that is a little low.

Lesson: The verbal response in this example may be
less effective than the silent response above. The
verbal response gives the opponent the information that,
although low, her offer seems to be in the ballpark.

Tempo

Silence can control the tempo of a negotiation and it
can shift the momentum from your opponent. This is
especially true when he makes a tactical or strategic
mistake.

Example 8.6
Hospital administrator: So, Dr. Smith, your salary
will be $150,000 a year.
Doctor: Fine.
Hospital administrator: You will have medical and
malpractice insurance.
Doctor: Good.
Hospital administrator: You will have four weeks
paid vacation.
Doctor: As we agreed.
Hospital administrator: You will be committing to
six years full time and then if you need extra time for
maternity leave or flex-time, we will work it out.
Doctor: (long silence)
Hospital administrator: (flustered, recognizing the
mistake) I didn't mean to imply that...obviously, under
the law...you are certainly within your rights to....

Doctor: (after another long pause and silence) Let's move on for now to life insurance, office space, and coverage terms.

Lesson: The physician used silence to communicate her intense displeasure at what was said. She has also effectively masked her future intentions and completely seized the control, power, and momentum of the negotiation. She will be more likely to gain concessions.

Conclusion

Recall the Miranda warnings a person receives when he or she is arrested. That language is, "You have the right to remain silent. Anything you say can and will be used against you." This is equally true in negotiations. Also remember the authors' advice: Anything you don't say can and will be used to benefit you.

Chapter 9 How to Gain
Valuable Concessions

Room to Negotiate

Concessions are an important part of any negotiation.
The first rule to remember is to leave yourself adequate
room to negotiate. This increases your flexibility. It
also gives you the ability to react to your opponent's
reasoning, facts, figures, and arguments. In short, you
can concede on certain points in order to get something
in return and to close the deal.

Example 9.1
Prospective employee: Your offer of $32,500 is low.
I would love to work with you, but I need $35,000.
Doctor: Well, I gave you all I had.... I guess I could
talk to my partners. We would hate to lose you for
$2,500.

Lesson: The doctor has left himself a little wiggle
room. He communicated that he may very well not go
any higher, but has left himself the option to agree after
talking to his partners.

Recognizing Concessions

In almost every negotiation there will come a time in
which you have to give up something to make progress.
It is crucially important, therefore, that you leave
yourself adequate room to negotiate. During your
preparation you should consider possible concessions

you might make, their cost to you, and their value to your opponent. When you give up *anything* during a negotiation, you are making a concession. This includes granting your opponent's request or yielding on a point. This also includes the situation where your opponent introduces a significant demand, unexpected request, or trial balloon. Your not dismissing it out of hand is a concession and should be viewed as such. You need to minimize what you give up (in terms of its cost to *you*) and maximize what you receive. At the same time, you should try to maintain or develop a good ongoing working relationship with your opponent.

Example 9.2
Opponent: This negotiation session is scheduled to go until 2:00 P.M. today. We cannot finish by 2:00. Can you stay until 4:00 P.M.?
Doctor: Okay.

Lesson: Everything you give up is a concession. The doctor has made a concession but has handled it poorly. He trivialized the value of his concession and has obtained nothing of value in return.

Example 9.3
Employee: My boyfriend is coming to the United States for three months. He is a talented computer specialist. Is there any chance you could hire him for the summer?
Doctor: As you know, we are not hiring. Money is tight, but get me his resume and I will consider it. I am making no promises. We need to square away your future employment here.

Employee: Thank you. I really appreciate your even considering him.

Lesson: Sometimes even a symbolic gesture can be a significant concession. It should be recognized as such.

Value

You need to understand the value of any concession to your opponent. The more valuable the concession, the more you can ask for and expect in return. The value that your opponent places on a concession will depend upon how badly she needs the concession, how hard you make her work for it, and the perceived cost to you. The most important thing to remember about concessions is that **what may be a crucial concession from your opponent's point of view may cost you little or nothing.** These are the concessions you should search for and use freely in your negotiation.

Example 9.4

Opponent: This negotiation session is scheduled to go until 2:00 P.M. today. Can you stay until 4:00 P.M.?
Doctor: Well, this was scheduled weeks ago. I would have to try and move things around. Do you want me to make a call to my office?
Opponent: If you can.
Doctor: (five minutes later) I changed the two appointments. I guess I will be working late again tonight.
Opponent: I appreciate it.
Doctor: (seizing the initiative) Now that we have a little breathing space, let's get to the salary issue.

Lesson: The doctor recognized the opponent's need for the extension, made her work for it, and clearly pointed out the cost of the concession to himself. He is now in a stronger position to obtain a concession from the opponent.

Example 9.5

You are writing a book and you know that it will be done on time. Your publisher struggles with chasing authors for their work and making up production and marketing schedules. Delay costs publishers money. What if you guarantee that your book will be done on time or early? This costs you nothing. To the publisher, it may be valued as a major concession. In return, you might ask for slightly higher royalties if delivered early.

Example 9.6

During the Arab-Israeli peace talks of the late 1970s, the handshake and photo opportunity of Menachem Begin and Anwar Sadat shaking hands was the lead story on the news across the world. This was a major concession from the Israeli point of view and was treated as such by all parties. The Israelis used this concession to their advantage.

Linkage

You should try to get something of equal or greater value in return for each concession you make. One of the most effective techniques for achieving this is *linkage*. The effective use of linkage requires that you evaluate and have your opponent evaluate each potential concession in the context of the entire proposed agreement. What at first blush seems very significant or insurmountable may, in the context of the big picture, be a relatively minor concession. Consider the following examples.

Example 9.7

Prospective employer: Doctor, we are looking for a three-year covenant not to compete within 100 miles of our office. Is that acceptable?

Doctor: No, it is not.

Prospective employer: What is the problem?

Doctor: I am a little taken aback by your lack of trust with the request for a three-year covenant not to compete. It doesn't bode well for a future relationship.

Prospective employer: (backpedaling and attempting to soften the blow) How could we make it work?

Doctor: If I was to get $160,000 for year one and $170,000 for year two, I would consider a 50-mile covenant not to compete.

Lesson: The physician linked his concession on the covenant not to compete with his demand for increased salary.

Example 9.8

Doctor: What I need is an additional $16,000 to sign this three-year contract for services.

Opponent: I can't do...

Doctor: Jim, we are talking about a $1.6 million contract, a staff member spread over three years. We have tailored the agreement for you. We only need 1% more to wrap this up. Let's not have to start negotiating from scratch.

Lesson: The doctor has emphasized the overall context in an effort to minimize the significance of his $16,000 demand.

Timing

You should always try to get your opponent to make the first major concession. This is true for the same reasons that you would want to get your opponent to make the first offer. The first major concession will frequently tip the negotiator's hand and reveal what she really wants. The concession may also reveal how badly she wants something and, in some cases, what she is willing to give up to get it. Making the first major concession is often perceived as a sign of weakness. Experienced negotiators can sense this weakness and will not hesitate to exploit it to the fullest extent.

Example 9.9
New doctor: We have been going back and forth for three hours. I asked for $90,000 and you offered $65,000. As you know, I have student loans, a family, and other expenses. My spouse is not working. I will drop my request to $80,000. I need to line up employment.
Practice leader: I appreciate your frankness. I am already over budget but I will talk to the powers that be and see if I can get you $72,500. Otherwise, if this is not satisfactory.... (putting papers in file)
Doctor: Thank you. I appreciate whatever you can do for me.

Lesson: By making the first major concession, the physician has lost power in the negotiation and revealed his desire to close the deal. He has also revealed his ability to accept $80,000. The opponent used this information against him.

Size and Rate of Concessions

You should start with the largest concession first and reduce the size of your concessions as the negotiation progresses. This technique is effective because of the emotional investment of your opponent as you get farther along in the negotiations. (See pages 108-109 on investment.) After hours, days, weeks, or months of negotiations, it becomes increasingly difficult, if not impossible, for your opponent to walk away from the potential deal. After you have positioned your opponent into this state of mind, it is time to reduce the size of your concessions.

Example 9.10
Health care officer: Kathy, we have been at this for four months. We wanted to purchase your practice. We started out at $1.5 million, went to $1.7 million, and then to $2 million.
Doctor: We have moved also. We went from $2.8 million to $2.6 million, down to $2.5 million.
Health care officer: We have been "moving" a lot more than you have.
Doctor: You have a lot more money than we have. Was your gross income $54 million last year?
Health care officer: Will you move off the $2.5 million?
Doctor: We might be able to.

Health care officer: Let's split the difference,[1] call it $2.25, and be done with it!

Doctor: We can't afford to split the difference. We can go to $2.4 million, bottom line. (getting out of chair)

Health care officer: Let me make a call.

Lesson: By holding fairly firm, the doctor was able to gain major concessions from the purchaser. She correctly determined that her opponent was heavily invested and would not want to walk away from the deal.

Information and Rate of Concessions

There is much information to be gleaned by the rate of concessions made by your opponent. An opponent who does not have to check with anyone has extensive authority. On the other hand, an opponent who must keep checking with others may in fact have limited authority. When the increments of concessions are increased as the negotiation progresses, this tells you that your opponent needs the deal more than you do. If you fall into a predictable pattern of concessions, you may tip off your opponent as to what your next concession will be.

Example 9.11
Doctor: (to owner of building) We can go to $260,000 for the building.
Owner: I can't do it for $260,000.
Doctor: How about $270,000?
Owner: You are getting closer.

---

[1] See pages 177-179 on splitting the difference.

Lesson: The owner will keep asking for more and more until the physician reaches his top dollar. A better response would have been, "What can you do it for?" The answer to that question might have been a number less than $270,000.

The Story of Concessions

Almost every opponent will report back to a boss or spouse regarding the negotiation. The story that your opponent reports is significant. This story will help justify the concessions made and will make your opponent look good or bad. Ideally, the story should be worded so that your opponent looks like a hero. You should interweave this potential story into the negotiation. You want your opponents to be able to visualize how they can sell the deal so their concessions come off looking good. The more concessions they can sell, the more they can give you.

Example 9.12
Your opponent leaves her office at 10:00 A.M., meets you at 10:05, and says that she will offer you $50,000 for your medical invention. You agree and she reports back to her boss at 10:15 and tells her the story.

Lesson: Your opponent's boss will say, "You should have offered less. You overpaid." The negotiation was concluded too quickly. There was no resistance. This may impede future negotiations.

Example 9.13
The same opponent as in Example 9.12 leaves the office at 10:00 A.M. and calls her boss at 2:00 P.M. to

say that negotiations are difficult. The doctor has read a negotiation book and is using everything he has learned. She staggers back to the office at 4:45 P.M. and goes through all the demands and problems, but says she got the signature for $52,500.

Lesson: The boss is likely to compliment your opponent because you were tough and the negotiation was hard fought and protracted. The experienced physician negotiator recognizes this need to report back and look good. When you acknowledge to your opponent that you are in the same boat and also have to look good, you develop an "us against them" negotiating relationship. Making your opponent look good is important if you will be negotiating with that person again in the future.

Chapter 10 Using and Breaking Deadlock

Appear Willing to Walk Away

The goal of negotiation is *not* to get an agreement. The goal is rather to reach an agreement that is favorable and meets your needs. Many physicians will agree to unfavorable terms to avoid a deadlock. Deadlock for these physicians has become synonymous with failure and is to be avoided at all costs. You should not fear deadlock. In fact, you should be able to use the anticipation of deadlock as a negotiating technique. **Most importantly, you need to be able to give the impression to the other side that you are prepared to walk away from the deal.**

Example 10.1
Attorney: Unless we are able to work out this new retainer agreement, our firm will not be able to continue to represent your medical group.
Doctor: I understand.
Attorney: Will you agree to our $250 per hour partner time, $175 per hour associate time, and $100 per hour paralegal time?
Doctor: As I mentioned previously, it is too high.
Attorney: I guess we are at an impasse.
Doctor: (calm and ignoring the last comment) How long will it take you to pull our files together and transfer them to the new firm, Cost-Yu-Less?
Attorney: Let's not be impetuous. I am sure we can work something out.

Lesson: The doctor did not agree to a bad deal just to get any deal. More importantly, by giving the impression that she was willing to walk away, the doctor will probably be able to gain concessions.

Break or Avoid Deadlock

In some cases you will want to attempt to break or avoid a deadlock. This can occur if you do not want to jeopardize an existing or potential long-term relationship. It can also occur when you need the deal and have few, if any, palatable alternatives. There are various methods you can use to avoid a deadlock. These include conciliatory language, flexibility, room to negotiate, cautious use of deadlines and ultimatums, eliminating the possibility of deadlocks, and "change" during the negotiation session.

CONCILIATORY LANGUAGE

If you feel close to an unwanted deadlock, a simple question or statement may help. It may even put the negotiation back on the right track.

Example 10.2

Provider: You want us to change our reimbursement for covered services and our payor alternative reimbursement schedule?

Doctor: Correct, we need the slight change to make it work for us.

Provider: No can do. We do not want to rewrite our standard agreement.

Doctor: We appreciate your prior movement and flexibility and your need to maintain a standard agreement. We are a unique facility. One fair way around the problem would be to attach an addendum to the contract. This would be fair to us and would still enable you to deal with your concerns.

Lesson: The doctor used conciliatory language, employed active listening skills (see pages 64-82 on active listening skills), stressed fairness, and offered a simple, cost-effective solution. Deadlock may be avoided.

FLEXIBILITY

The successful physician negotiator has carefully prepared for the negotiation (see pages 117-132 on preparation) and has built flexibility into his or her decision tree (see pages 112-113 on flexibility). Flexibility may be needed to avoid deadlock.

Example 10.3
Prospective employer: (after extensive negotiations) We would love to have you on board, but the most we can offer for salary is $130,000 and, as I understand it, you need $150,000.
Doctor: That's right.
Prospective employer: I wish I could come up with the $20,000, but my hands are tied. We have a salary structure.
Doctor: If I take the $130,000 and am allowed to retain any money I can generate from trauma call, honoraria, royalties, IMEs, and occasionally testifying as an expert witness....
Prospective employer: As long as it does not interfere with your duties. That works for me.

Lesson: The physician used flexibility and her ability as a problem solver to avoid an unwanted deadlock.

The concession was granted because it cost the employer little if anything.

ADEQUATE ROOM TO NEGOTIATE

Leaving adequate room to negotiate will help avoid most deadlocks. (See page 139 on room to negotiate.) As part of your preparation, you should "play out" the negotiation scenario by working backwards from the desired goal to the starting point. You need to understand and anticipate your opponent's desires, goals, needs, and likely reaction to offers. An adequate physician negotiator reacts well to offers and demands. The sophisticated negotiator will also be able to plan the negotiation so that an opponent will almost have to make the desired concessions.

Example 10.4

Prospective employer: We are getting close to an agreement. The salary is $150,000 plus a bonus.

Doctor: I need assurances that the practice will be growing and thriving and will not be in financial difficulty like my last practice. What kind of growth are you looking at?

Prospective employer: We anticipate an increase in revenue of $450,000 after you sign on for year one, and $500,000 for year two.

Doctor: I am looking for a 7% bonus on the increase in gross revenue on a consolidated basis, with the right to withhold consent for capitated and reduced contracts, post-termination collections for two years, with a guaranteed base bonus amount of $30,000 for year one and $32,000 for year two.

Prospective employer: (taken aback somewhat) I see you have done your homework. However, we can only go to 5%, and about the guaranteed base bonus....

Lesson: When your opponent is attempting to sell an overly optimistic picture with what you consider to be inflated future projections, you can make those numbers work for you while at the same time leaving yourself room to negotiate. Savvy physician negotiators induce their opponents to come up with these rosy, or in some cases, inflated, projections. They then anchor their demands on these projections. It is difficult, if not impossible, when the above is done correctly, for your opponents to move away from these numbers. After all *they* are the ones that offered them in the first place.

DEADLINES AND ULTIMATUMS

Hard and fast ultimatums and "drop-dead" deadlines (see pages 92-102 on deadlines) can quickly lead to deadlock. They represent inflexibility and may leave you little room to negotiate. The most effective ultimatums and deadlines are ones that deliver the message without completely cutting off the possibility of continued negotiations. Here is where knowing your opponent and the right buttons to push become crucial. (See pages 123-124 on knowing your opponent.)

Example 10.5
Doctor: Unless you agree to sign this two-year covenant not to compete, we cannot hire you!
Prospective employee: (angrily offering his hand) Thank you for your time!

Lesson: The doctor's statement left him no room to negotiate. If his bluff is called, he has lost the opportunity to make a new hire.

Example 10.6
Doctor: Tell me what it is like to be an All-American football player.
Prospective employee: A lot of hard work, but the scholarship paid my way all through school and I made a lot of great friends on the team. I am still close to....
Doctor: How many colleges were after you?
Prospective employee: Fifteen or twenty.
Doctor: What made you go to BC?
Prospective employee: It is a great school—great team, good academics—and it was around the Flutie era.
Doctor: That's what we have here; a "great team," excellent medicine. We need you to sign a letter of intent just like you did at BC. We need a level of commitment. The covenant not to compete is our assurance that you will not "jump to Notre Dame" the first chance you get. Are you a team player, Jim?
Prospective employee: Yes, I am.
Doctor: Let's get this contract signed and work on your position on the team.

Lesson: The doctor was able to get the covenant not to compete by pushing his opponent's buttons and attacking around his opponent's flank. He avoided a frontal assault and did not make any take it or leave it demands that may have backfired.

ELIMINATING THE POSSIBILITY OF DEADLOCK

The best way to deal with the specter of deadlock is to eliminate it completely. If you can get your opponent to agree that deadlock is not an option, you have gone a long way to eliminate the possibility of deadlock. This requires recognition by both parties that they *need* to avoid a deadlock and to reach an agreement. The sophisticated physician negotiator will plant the seeds for this type of commitment early on in the negotiation in case it is needed later.

Example 10.7

Doctor: Are you really committed to reaching an agreement on the terms of this contract?

Opponent: I have the same level of commitment to reaching an agreement that you have.

Doctor: I am willing to cancel the rest of the day and my dinner plans and agree to stay in this room with you until we reach an agreement.

Opponent: Agreed. Let's take five minutes to make some calls and get back to work.

Lesson: The agreement to avoid a deadlock was made well in advance. Although this agreement is not binding, it will be helpful in avoiding a deadlock.

Example 10.8

Doctor: Nancy, we have been negotiating for two hours. You have looked at your watch four times and taken three calls on your cell phone. Are you sure you have time to reach a fair agreement *today*?

Opponent: That's why I came to your office—to reach an agreement.

Doctor: I am willing to cancel out and agree to stay in this room until we reach an agreement.

Opponent: Agreed. Let's take five minutes.

Lesson: The opponent has been positioned to buy into the concept of closure.

CHANGE

Physicians need to recognize when a negotiation is heading for an unwanted deadlock. You can use change to avoid the deadlock. A change in the time frame, location, goals, negotiator, and type of negotiation can help avoid an unwanted deadlock.

Example 10.9
Doctor: It doesn't look like we will be able to give each one of the issues you raised adequate discussion time today. I suggest that we schedule another session to complete the job so we are not rushed.
Opponent: Agreed. How does Tuesday at 2:00 P.M. work for you?

Lesson: Putting the issue over to another negotiating session is one way to avoid a deadlock. You and your opponent may have different views during the new session. In addition, circumstances for either party may have changed in the interim.

Example 10.10
Doctor: I feel uncomfortable in this setting. Your staff keeps interrupting us and the noise.... What if we continue this in a nice, quiet, neutral environment? I could call and get us a conference room two blocks from here where we will not be interrupted. I think we will make more progress over there.
Prospective employer: (reluctantly) Well, let me pack up my stuff and tell my staff where I will be.

Lesson: The change of location may help facilitate the negotiation.

Part of being a flexible negotiator is being able to roll with the punches. If it becomes apparent that you will not be able to reach the goal you originally intended, you may want to modify your goal so as not to come away empty handed. Caution: Do not fall into the trap of being so invested in the negotiation process that you agree to almost anything to avoid coming away without a deal. (See pages 108-109 on investment.) There is nothing wrong, however, with modifying or scaling back your goal so long as the agreement reached still is favorable to you.

Example 10.11
Doctor: What we are looking for is $24,000 a year to write and edit your new medical-legal newsletter.
Publisher: We can't commit that kind of money. What if the newsletter does not take off?
Doctor: We are confident it will do well. It will fill a much-needed niche. We will agree to write and edit the newsletter on a monthly basis for $2,000 a month with a 60-day notice to discontinue.
Publisher: Make it a 30-day notice to discontinue and you have a deal.

Lesson: The doctor employed the technique of gradualism to salvage a deal headed toward deadlock. While she didn't achieve her original goal, she did achieve favorable terms. Once the newsletter catches on, another attempt can be made to get a longer commitment.

Sometimes negotiation deadlock can be broken by employing a new negotiator. This technique requires an admission that someone else may be more likely to avoid a deadlock. An admission that they may not be the best person to achieve a favorable agreement is difficult for many physicians. You must recognize that passing a negotiation to a partner or colleague is not an admission of failure. When there is someone else in a better position to score, it is time to pass the ball. Sometimes the mere suggestion that you may have to change negotiators can itself be used to help avoid a deadlock. Your opponent will be concerned with having to start over and/or dealing with someone who is even more difficult.

Example 10.12
Doctor: We are not really making any progress, are we?
Computer salesperson: We are not. I have tried to explain to you the merits...cost savings...how the system will work for you and not cost you....
Doctor: The problem is that I am probably not the right person to talk to. Let me get Dr. Patton. You two will be able to talk "computerese" without much of the translating you were doing for me.
Computer salesperson: Is she available now?

Lesson: A deadlock has been avoided. Dr. Patton's computer knowledge may help facilitate the process. The doctor was sophisticated enough to realize that turning the process over to Dr. Patton may be helpful and should not be seen as a sign of failure.

Example 10.13
Doctor: I know we have been at this for three hours, but the bottom line is that the $74,000 price is a sticking point.

Computer salesperson: That's the best we can do.
Doctor: Maybe I am completely off-base here. You might be better off if you start *fresh* with my partner, Dr. Hardass. She knows a lot about computers. She is tough but fair. Don't be put off by her abrasive manner....
Computer salesperson: I would rather resolve this with you right now. If I made a call and knocked 10% off the top....

Lesson: The very mention of starting over with a new negotiator has strengthened the doctor's position.

To avoid a deadlock, the sophisticated physician negotiator will rapidly change the type of negotiation while it is in progress. Changing a competitive negotiation into a cooperative one is particularly helpful. (See pages 12-23 on competitive and cooperative negotiations.)

Example 10.14
Doctor: Let's forget about my demands for a moment and concentrate on what additional items, terms, or conditions we could add or modify to make this a win-win situation for both of us. Let's stop discussing how to split up the pie and let's concentrate on making a bigger pie where there is plenty for both of us. What do you say?
Opponent: It sounds good to me. If you could....

Lesson: The doctor changed a competitive negotiation to a cooperative one to avoid an unwanted deadlock.

<u>Conclusion</u>

The successful physician negotiator will not fear deadlock, but will use the potential for deadlock as an offensive negotiation technique. The use of conciliatory language, flexibility, adequate room to negotiate, deadlines and ultimatums, eliminating the possibility of deadlock, and change are all methods to avoid or to move away from an unwanted deadlock. Remember, you need to be prepared to walk away from a deal. This is particularly true when you have a better alternative, if the deal does not meet your needs, when you may be able to get a better agreement at a later time from your opponent, or when the deal violates your professional or personal morals or ethics. Under these circumstances, the deadlock is not unwanted and you should walk away from the proposed agreement.

Chapter 11 Using Controlled Emotions to Your Advantage

Emotions can play a key role in negotiations. You need to understand how to use emotions to your advantage. Techniques using emotions include playing it cool, controlling anger, personalizing, and tapping into the fear or anxiety of an opponent. These techniques are discussed below.

Playing It Cool

You will sometimes be faced with an opponent who is getting agitated, screaming, or yelling. Your natural reaction is to assume that your opponent probably has a valid point or he or she wouldn't be screaming. This is a flawed assumption. You need to remember that just because someone is yelling and screaming does not mean that they are right.

It is equally important to try not to lose your temper during a negotiation. Losing your temper could easily result in your saying or doing something that you might later regret. If you feel you are getting close to the edge, ask for and take a break. (See pages 205-207 on taking a break.)

Example 11.1

Lawyer: (to doctor's assistant, talking in a loud, threatening voice) The doctor is in big trouble. I am in court. The case is coming up in one hour. The doctor did not fill out the medical-legal report. We ordered it two weeks ago. We will now lose the case. The client will have every right to look to the doctor for damages because of her failure to fill out the report.

Doctor's assistant: Is there anything we can do?

Lawyer: Yes, I will send the client over in a half hour to pick up the report. Get the doctor. Make her sit down and dictate the report and type it up. If you can give the client three copies I will try and postpone the case for one hour. This could solve the doctor's problem.

Doctor's assistant: Okay. We will get right on it. Sorry for the trouble.

Lesson: In this true example, the attorney had *not* previously sent the request to the doctor's office. The attorney used a loud and threatening manner to bully the doctor to help him. The moral of this example is that just because someone is yelling and screaming about a particular point in a negotiation does not make the person right.

DIFFUSING THE OPPONENT

When faced with an emotional opponent, you should attempt to sift through his or her emotions to the substance of the person's position. One technique for accomplishing this is to move the opponent from the general to the specific. This will focus the energy of the negotiation on the relevant issues and will help determine how justified, if at all, your opponent's strong emotions really are.

Example 11.2

Opponent: (to doctor, yelling) Your proposal is outrageous. I should just get up and walk out of here. I have never been so insulted in all of my professional career.

Doctor: (in control) I can see you are not happy. Let's take the four key points one at a time and see if we can't get some closure. Okay, on issue number 1....

Lesson: What the doctor is really trying to drive home is that as long as the opponent is yelling and screaming, he can't really "hear her." By moving to the specific, he will be able to determine if his opponent's anger is at all justified.

Controlling Your Anger

Emotions that are released in a calculated and controlled manner can be helpful. When you feel that your opponent has crossed the line and said something totally inappropriate, it is legitimate for you to get angry. The key is not to go off the deep end with your anger. If you do, you could reveal damaging information or say something that would permanently destroy your working relationship with your opponent.

Example 11.3
Colleague: The reason we are having financial trouble is because of questionable medical competency.
Doctor: That's bullshit and you know it. I don't have to take this shit. How dare you question my competency.
Colleague: I'm sorry, I didn't mean to imply that you weren't competent. Look, we'll find the money for your raise. Again, my deepest apologies.

Lesson: The doctor has used controlled anger to pounce on a point. This use of anger may help him gain power in, and seize the momentum of, the negotiation.

PERSONALIZE THE NEGOTIATION

Personalizing the negotiation may be helpful. People are generally nice and like helping other people out. On the other hand, people generally couldn't care less about helping out a corporation or other business entity. When you personalize the negotiation, you tap into your opponent's natural desire to help another person out. The successful physician negotiator attempts to make each negotiation personal, rather than a negotiation between corporate conglomerates. When this is done, you will be more likely to obtain concessions. If the person you are negotiating with likes you, then personalizing the negotiation is that much more effective. (See pages 79-80 on your opponent liking you.) Note that there is nothing wrong with asking for a personal favor as long as you do not overuse this technique. Consider the following examples.

Example 11.4
Doctor: I will get to the chart dictation as soon as I can.
Medical records charge nurse: You don't really appreciate the situation. I need this done *today*. My credibility is on the line.
Doctor: You are taking this much too personally.
Medical records charge nurse: I have to take it personally. My job is on the line.
Doctor: I'll see what I can do.

Lesson: People generally do not like to see other people lose their jobs. This is because they would never want to lose their own job and thus have compassion for the other person. Here the nurse

164

effectively personalized the negotiation and used the doctor's compassion to her advantage.

Example 11.5

Doctor: (to long-time opponent) Just this one time, as a personal favor, I need you to.... I will not forget it.

Lesson: The opponent may very well concede. He may be thinking of the time in the future when he really needs to get something for himself. At that point he may be asking for a quid pro quo.

Example 11.6

Doctor: I need to obtain the change in the lease that we talked about.
Leasing agent: We did not officially offer that change.
Doctor: Based on your representation, I already told my employer about the change. If you backpedal on this, I am in big trouble.
Leasing agent: Let me work something out.

Lesson: Everyone can relate to getting in trouble with a boss. Use of this threat to yourself can gain you sympathy and concessions from your opponent.

Tapping into Fear or Anxiety

You should use your opponents' fears and anxieties against them. Before you can use these fears, you need to understand what they are. (See pages 95-96 on fear and anxiety.) Common fears you can use against your opponent are the fears of failure, loss, and embarrassment. Consider the following examples.

Example 11.7
Doctor: What are you going to do if we are not able to negotiate an agreement on the terms of your contract?
Prospective employee: Well, I guess I will continue to send out my CV. I do have some other feelers out there.

Lesson: The negative consequences of failure have been put in the mind of the opponent. This should make it psychologically easier for the opponent to grant concessions to avoid failure. Even asking innocent questions such as, "What will happen if you don't bring back an agreement?" can raise the anxiety level of your opponent.

Example 11.8
Doctor: How many claims are you handling currently?
Insurance adjuster: Two hundred forty-seven.
Doctor: (sympathetically) That's a lot of claims. With that many cases there must be a lot of pressure to resolve them and move on.
Insurance adjuster: I get seven to ten new ones each week.
Doctor: It's Friday. How many have you adjusted this week?
Insurance adjuster: Three, not counting this one.
Doctor: You are losing ground. My good friend was an adjuster. I went up to see him one day and the company had a big GOYA chart on the wall.
Insurance adjuster: GOYA?
Doctor: Yes, Get Off Your Ass (GOYA). They charted the number of cases each adjuster settled and posted the results. Should we try and resolve my claim or should I send a note to the company and tell them we couldn't work it out and put it into litigation?

Insurance adjuster: Let's keep talking.

Lesson: In some cases, the fear or anxiety is not expressly mentioned, but is subtly talked around. This can be even more effective because it may be harder for your opponent to detect that she is the target of a negotiation tactic.

Example 11.9
Experienced attorney: This is a straightforward workers' compensation case. The claimant fell at work, triggering her multiple sclerosis. Here are the medical reports on causation and disability.
Novice: Which side of the courtroom should I stand on?
Experienced attorney: Here on the left, furthest from the workers' compensation judge. One point—because you do not have a medical report, when she asks you what you have to say, I wouldn't say too much, just that you are opposing the request, and sit down. You don't want to embarrass yourself.
Novice: Thank you.

Lesson: The fear of being embarrassed is one that can be used effectively by the sophisticated physician negotiator. Your opponent, whether a doctor, lawyer, or other professional, especially if he or she is inexperienced or a novice, may go to great lengths to avoid personal or professional embarrassment. This example is true. The injured worker was placed on workers' compensation for multiple sclerosis due to the trauma of a fall. The fear of embarrassment played a significant role in the pre-hearing negotiation between the experienced and the novice attorney. This type of negotiation is played out routinely at the expense of inexperienced or novice negotiators.

Conclusion

You need to be able to play it cool and control your emotions. You should understand that just because people are yelling and screaming does not make them right. Take your opponent's emotional objections from the general to the specific and use the controlled anger technique when appropriate. Personalize the negotiation and occasionally ask for personal favors. Finally, understand and capitalize on your opponent's fears and anxieties.

Chapter 12 Telephone Negotiations

At least twenty to sixty percent of your negotiations will be conducted over the telephone. There are methods that you can use to gain an advantage during telephone negotiations. These methods include focusing, preparing, initiating the call, setting the agenda, listening for auditory feedback, taking notes, and sending the confirmation letter. Each of these methods is discussed below.

Concentrate and Focus

Telephone negotiations can be just as important as in-person negotiations. A negotiation that may have taken hours in person may take only minutes or even seconds over the phone. When things happen that quickly, you really need to force yourself to focus on the negotiation. You must recognize the importance of focusing on your telephone negotiation. Failure to do so can be disastrous.

Example 12.1
Computer salesperson: Doctor, the service agreement for your computer equipment is running out at the end of the week. Should I put you down for the two-year renewal? The cost is the same.
Doctor: Fine, send along the paperwork.

Lesson: The accelerated pace of phone call negotiations can result in the physician not negotiating at all. Even when one or both of the parties has the time to negotiate (see pages 83-87 on time), the result of these "quickie" negotiations can be extreme—with one party winning and one party losing.

Example 12.2
Doctor: Busy?
Colleague: Swamped!
Doctor: Me, too. I will be lucky if I get out of here by 8:00 tonight. Did you look at our proposed lease? $3,500 a month and you are in our new building.
Colleague: $2,000 a month for year one and $2,500 for years two to four.
Doctor: Done. I will have my attorney send over the lease.

Lesson: Here the doctor conducted a negotiation involving thousands of dollars in seconds. Had he taken more time, he would have saved a substantial amount of money.

Prepare

Telephone negotiations happen quickly. When dealing with such fast-paced negotiations, you need to be fully prepared and organized. You need to have your facts, figures, files, research notes, documents, computer, calculator, and other materials organized and ready to be used quickly and efficiently. Many negotiations are lost due to the inability of the negotiator to put her hands on a crucial file or piece of paper.

Example 12.3
Provider: We can offer you $2,400 for your
outstanding bill of $4,900. This is a one-time offer. Is
that acceptable?
Doctor: That's less than 50%! Joanne, can you get me
that file? This was a difficult and complex case!
Provider: Doctor, we have been through this with your
billing clerk already. Your provider agreement clearly
states....
Doctor: (rummaging through file) I think we called
you for authorization before.... If I could only find that
phone message. These little pink slips drive me crazy!

Lesson: The doctor needed to be better prepared. If he
was, he would have had the information readily
available. If he cannot find the missing document, he
should suspend the negotiation and call the provider
back after he does locate it.

Initiate the Call

The party who originates the call is at a distinct
advantage. She has time to prepare, is not taken off
guard, can prepare a checklist, and can organize the key
files and documents. The initiating party will also be
able to select a quiet time and a place free of
distractions to make the call from. If you initiate the
call and catch your opponent "cold," your opponent's
surprise and lack of preparation can work in your favor.
You can also use your initiation of the call as an
opportunity to set the agenda and thus control the issues
to be discussed.

You will need to be able to defend against this
tactic when you receive a call. First you need to listen
carefully for the purpose of the call. Once you
recognize the call as the start of a negotiation, you

should obtain as much information as you can. You should then call the party back at a convenient time when you can properly prepare yourself.

Example 12.4
Opponent: Hi, doctor. How are you?
Doctor: (doing two things in addition to talking on phone) Busy.
Opponent: Let me get right to business then. I am calling to discuss the buyout provision of your equipment lease.
Doctor: When is the lease up? How much is the proposed buyout in the contract? What specifically are you looking for?
Opponent: The lease is up at the end of the month. There is no specific amount mentioned, just the "resale value," but we are looking for $24,000 and the equipment is yours free and clear!
Doctor: I will get back to you later this week. I will pull my file, talk to my office manager, and see if we even want this equipment. It is, after all, three years old. I will call you.

Lesson: The doctor recognized the importance of the pending telephone negotiation. She correctly gathered as much information as possible and stated that she would call her opponent back.

Example 12.5
Doctor: (to prospective employee) This is a call to see if we can wrap up the loose ends of your taking the position. I need to get closure on three issues: salary, starting date, and hospital coverage. On the salary, the offer on the table is $130,000. Is that acceptable?

Lesson: The doctor did not ask if this was a convenient time, nor did he ask if the prospective employee had any issues to add to the agenda. The doctor used his initiation of the call as a way to control the agenda and resolve the issues that he wanted to resolve.

Listen for Auditory Feedback

Telephone negotiations do not allow you to read your opponent's body language (see pages 71-74 on body language) and other nonverbal communication. Many opponents will find it much easier to say no over the phone than in person. This is the reason why some experts recommend limiting your phone negotiations to those situations where you suspect that *you* will be saying no. The realities of the workplace make it difficult, if not impossible, to avoid telephone negotiations. Few, if any, physicians are able to fly 3,000 miles to conduct a ten-minute negotiation in person.

The only information you receive from your opponent during a telephone negotiation is auditory information. You need to be very sensitive to this auditory feedback. Active listening is required. (See pages 64-82 on active listening.) The pitch, tone, volume, pauses, topic selection, silences, and other auditory cues are your only sources of information. Some experienced negotiators go so far as to close their eyes so they can better concentrate on what is and is not being verbalized.

Example 12.6
Doctor: How does that proposal sound?
Opponent: Well, generally, it sounds good. (long pause)
Doctor: I sense your hesitation. Tell me what you are concerned about. As you know, we are looking for a long-term business relationship. We want to give you the best agreement we can.
Opponent: I have three major concerns.

Lesson: The doctor was able to sense her opponent's concerns. This is important because the doctor is looking for a win-win deal that will serve as the basis of a long-standing relationship.

Take Notes and Send Confirmation Letters

Telephone negotiations can result in many misunderstandings between the parties. You will need to take legible, comprehensive notes during telephone negotiations. To avoid problems with handwriting, it is best to have your notes typed/transcribed after the negotiation. Taking notes is also an opportunity for you to clarify your opponent's proposal during the negotiation.

You should consider turning your written notes into a memorandum of agreement and sending it to your opponent after the negotiation. The drafting of this memorandum is yet another opportunity to specify the terms of the deal, remove (and control) any ambiguities, and ensure that any oral assurances are specified in writing. For complex or significant agreements or those involving substantial amounts of money, you should consult with counsel *before* sending out the memorandum or agreement.

Example 12.7
Doctor: (to opponent) I want to write this down correctly. As I understand it, what you are offering is two years of free service and, if we agree today, you will throw in.... Is that correct?

Lesson: By summarizing his opponent's proposal, the physician has eliminated possible ambiguities and pinned his opponent down.

Conclusion

You need to recognize the need to prepare for telephone negotiations as if they were important face-to-face negotiations. Initiating the phone call can be helpful. It is important not to negotiate when you are not prepared. You should have all your tools readily accessible, set the agenda, and listen actively for auditory feedback. To make sure that there are no ambiguities, your notes should be converted into a letter to be sent to your opponent after the negotiation.

Chapter 13 Defeating Your Opponent's Tactics

Physicians must be able to "diagnose" and "treat" the myriad of negotiation tactics used by their opponents. Treatment is possible only when you are properly prepared. This chapter is designed to help you prepare to deal with your opponent's tactics. The negotiation tactics most frequently employed against physicians are discussed in the following sections.

Tactic 1: Let's Split the Difference

DIAGNOSIS

This tactic is usually fairly simple to diagnose. The proponent will suggest, "in the spirit of fairness and equity," that each side offer an equal concession in order to achieve a rapid conclusion to the negotiation. This request has a lot of surface appeal and is difficult, if not impossible, for most physician negotiators to resist. In the end, the negotiation tactic of an equal compromise is difficult to turn down. More money and other negotiables are lost due to this tactic than almost any other single tactic. When your opponent says to you, "Let's split the difference," what she is really saying is, "I want a 50% concession." Because this is a request for a major concession, it should be considered as carefully and cautiously as any other request for a concession. (See pages 139-148 on concessions.) The response you make to the tactic will usually determine the outcome of the negotiation.

Example 13.1
Opponent: (to doctor) Doctor, you were looking for $30,000 for your boat. I offered you $20,000. Let's split the difference and call it $25,000.

Lesson: This statement needs to be diagnosed as a demand for a 50% concession. Such a demand needs a careful response.

TREATMENT
A strong, reassured response can effectively neutralize the tactic without harming an existing or anticipated long-term relationship.

Example 13.2
Doctor: (to prospective new doctor) Fred, we can meet most of your terms with regard to insurance, coverage, staff, hours, and vacations. The final stumbling block is starting salary. You asked for $140,000 and we offered $120,000. We are willing to meet you half way and I am authorized to split the difference and go to $130,000. (offers his hand)
Fred: I wish I could split the difference, but I just cannot afford to with student loans, mortgages, a child on the way.... We did our budget....

Lesson: This was a direct rebuttal. It was possible because Fred was prepared to justify why he *required* $140,000. Fred refused to give in, but has left himself very little room to negotiate. The sophisticated physician negotiator would have anticipated the use of this tactic by an opponent and left himself more room to negotiate. (See page 139 on room to negotiate.)

Example 13.3
Doctor: (to prospective employee) Fred, I certainly understand about obligations. I do have to go back to my partners. If you can't split the difference, what can you do for us?
Fred: We might be able to make it on $138,000. I would want to check with my spouse before committing to that.

Lesson: The experienced physician negotiator reasonably anticipates the follow-up request after a refusal to split the difference. The concession he offered was less than what his opponent had demanded. The above response/concession may be made in order to foster a new long-term relationship and/or to get closure on the negotiation.

Example 13.4
Fred: I probably did not make myself clear and I am sorry. I cannot afford to posture or play games. The $140,000 is my bottom line. I know for the practice $2,000 or $3,000 is not a lot of money, but for us, it is make it or break it.

Lesson: Standing firm (with adequate justification) is an option. Because you have not left yourself any room to negotiate, you should only employ this tactic if you are prepared to walk away from the deal.

Tactic 2: Take It or Leave It

DIAGNOSIS
This is usually a simple tactic to recognize. The proponent will make an offer or demand and make it clear that this is her best offer and it is not negotiable.

When faced with this hardball tactic, many physicians will accept the dictated terms and not challenge their opponent's rationale or reasonableness. (See pages x-xi on the world's quickest negotiation.) You should not cave in to this type of pressure no matter how strongly this tactic is expressed. You should keep in mind your other alternatives.

Example 13.5
Attorney: We are sorry to see that you have been sued for medical malpractice for an amount exceeding your coverage. We would be pleased to defend you. We will need a $10,000 retainer and our hourly rate will be $300 an hour. (See pages 217-234 on negotiating and retaining an attorney.)
Doctor: I would like to talk about the retainer and the hourly rate.
Attorney: (cutting her off, pleasant but firm) Our rates have been set by the management committee. They are nonnegotiable.

Lesson: The message in the above example is clear (although not expressed in these exact words): *Take it or leave it!*

TREATMENT
You will need to recognize that take it or leave it is a hardball tactic and respond accordingly. What your opponent is really saying is: "I have all the power in this negotiation and will do and charge whatever I want!" The first thing you need to do is to evaluate the offer on its merits. You should not automatically accept or reject the offer. If you do not decide to reject it, you will need to neutralize the tactic. One good way to do this is to change the balance of power as quickly

and as painlessly as possible. This can be accomplished by stressing the desire to establish a long-term relationship.

Example 13.6
Doctor: (to attorney) As I was starting to say, we are looking for a firm to represent doctors in my situation. I will be the first case. I will be reporting back to the association, which has many doctors in similar situations. We are looking for a contract with a firm where there is a modest retainer against time— $2,500—and hourly rates for paralegals, associates, and partners. Should I be talking to you about this or one of the senior partners?

Lesson: By stressing the desire to begin a long-term relationship, the doctor has gained power in the negotiation.

You will also need to be prepared to walk away. As we have seen, the ability and determination to just say no is an absolute requirement if you want to be a successful physician negotiator. *Before* you do walk away, however, you need to be sure of what your alternatives are.

Example 13.7
Salesman: We've been going over this for thirty minutes. The price is $5,000, take it or leave it.
Doctor: Thanks for your time, I'll leave it. I can get comparable equipment for less than that. Can you find your own way out?

Salesman: Well, I think we'll still be able to work something out, how about $4,500?

Lesson: You need to be prepared to "leave it." This doctor knew that she could get comparable equipment for less than $5,000 and was therefore empowered to be able to decline her opponent's demand. Also, calling her opponent's bluff with the take it or leave it tactic was successful in gaining a major price concession. She was able to respond in this direct way *because she had alternatives.*

You should react to each take it or leave it proposal on its merits and not assume that just because it is the first offer, it is not a reasonable or fair one. You should be able to recognize and capitalize on many situations in which you can avoid unwanted and/or protracted negotiations through the use of a fair preemptive offer at the start of a negotiation. This variation of the take it or leave it technique is particularly effective when used before a negotiation starts. Use of this technique will save you the trouble and uncertainty of lengthy negotiations and can help to build trust in long-term relationships.

Example 13.8
Doctor: You have done an excellent job these past ten months. Rather than wait for your annual review, we are going to raise your salary by 10% effective the first of the month.
Office manager: Thank you.

Lesson: This preemptive, fair but firm offer combines the element of surprise with a softer version of take it or leave it. Through its use the doctor was able to avoid protracted negotiations, control the outcome, and build trust in her long-term relationship with her office manager.

Tactic 3: The Estimate: Ballpark Price

DIAGNOSIS

This tactic may be difficult to diagnose. It can be expressed in many ways and disguised quite successfully. Physicians, in their eagerness to help and desire to be liked, are particularly susceptible to this tactic. When this tactic is used, you will be asked for a rough estimate of the cost, time, and effort involved in a project soon to be a matter of negotiation. This rough estimate request is a very effective negotiation tactic. The proponent of the question is seeking the most crucial information of the negotiation; that is, the information to determine what is a fair price for the proposed work. Most importantly, the tactic serves to trap you into setting a price without adequate thought or analysis. (See pages 27-31 on ambush negotiations.) You may be assured that your opponent is just looking for a rough estimate and that no one will hold you to the price or terms. Do not fall into this trap. Once you have given an estimated price, it may be very difficult, if not impossible, to distance yourself from that price. Even when you are able to move away from the original figure, it is unlikely that you will reach the result that could have been achieved had you not been tied to the estimate. That is why the savvy opponent will frequently push you hard for your estimate. Consider the following examples where this tactic is employed.

Example 13.9
Opponent: (to doctor) Give me a rough estimate of how long it will take you to do the medical review for our CD-ROM project.

Example 13.10
Publisher: (to doctor) Doctor, approximately how much would you charge to edit our medical newsletter?

Example 13.11
Insurer: (to doctor) Doctor, how difficult will it be for you to set up protocol for our return-to-work program for our carpal tunnel syndrome employees?

Example 13.12
Insurance company executive: We admire your work in occupational medicine. We know you pride yourself on your efficiency. I have files I would like you to review. It is the first of what we hope will be a lot of new work. I would like to send you the file to review.
Doctor: That would be fine.
Insurance company executive: Would $500 be reasonable?
Doctor: Yes, send it along. How many other files do you have?

One week later...
Doctor: A messenger just delivered your records. The box weighs 43 pounds. You never mentioned the voluminous nature of the case!
Insurer: You never asked.
Doctor: I can't review this file for $500 and do a good and thorough job.

Insurer: Well, doctor, I already noted on the file that you agreed on $500. This puts me in an awkward position. We assumed that once you gave your word.... But as an accommodation, I will put an additional $250 on the file. You will get $750.00. Okay?

Doctor: Thank you.

Lesson: The doctor ends up thanking his opponent for paying him about 20% of what a fair price should be. She made a fatal error by agreeing to a price before knowing all the pertinent information. To avoid this problem in a consulting situation you should charge by the hour.

TREATMENT

As a preliminary matter, you need to be able to diagnose this tactic no matter how well it is disguised. You need to insist on being provided *all* of the details of the assignment before even attempting to start to estimate the time and effort or cost involved. Even then, you should proceed cautiously because it is difficult to retract statements once they are made. You need to appreciate that once a figure is placed on the table, it is often difficult, if not impossible, to move away from it.

Example 13.13

Corporate executive: We would like you to do three days of consulting work. Give me a ballpark figure on the cost. We will not hold you to it. I am putting my pen down. I will not even write your answer down.

Doctor: It will depend on the details of the assignment. What is the type of work to be done? Where is it to be done? How soon do you need the results? Why is the work being done?

Executive: Well, it is actually a rush job…. We need you to go to Chernobyl this August. It will be fieldwork but not too close to the meltdown. The U.S. government has contracted with us to do this work to see if we can help clean up the radiation any quicker. There are just too many people dying due to the radiation.

Doctor: Just out of curiosity, what is the dollar value of the contract you have received from the government?

Executive: It is a big job. But the total contract is $210 million.

Lesson: As you can see, frequently the devil is in the details. The doctor was well advised to obtain all the details of the assignment before giving *any* estimate as to the cost. If she had just jumped in and said that her consulting fee is $2,500 a day she probably would have not been able to successfully free herself from that quick estimate and negotiate a better deal for herself.

Tactic 4: Lack of Candor

DIAGNOSIS

This tactic is frequently difficult to diagnose. Your opponent may be shading the truth, not telling you the full truth, failing to correct false impressions you have, or, in fact, lying to you. While we would all like to think that everyone we are negotiating with is telling the full truth, we know that this is not the case. As a matter of fact, the legal system even permits salespeople and others to engage in "puffery" as an accepted business tactic. Thus, many opponents will not even have a legal obligation to tell the truth during negotiations. The sophisticated physician negotiator understands puffery and discounts much of what her opponent tells her.

You need to investigate, research, and fully prepare for your negotiation. (See pages 117-132 on preparation.) The diagnosis of lack of candor is made when the physician catches the opponent in misrepresentations or untruths. This can be verified by research conducted before the negotiation. You should also make a provisional diagnosis of lack of candor when you have a gut reaction or an instinctive feeling that an opponent is not being candid. Consider the following examples.

Example 13.14
Salesperson: (to doctor) That is a bottom-line price on the condo. There is no room to negotiate. A young couple is coming back today to sign a purchase and sale agreement.

Lesson: A classic ploy. You should immediately have a gut reaction that the salesperson is not being candid when he states that someone else is coming later to buy the property. If they liked it so much, why didn't they already buy it?

Example 13.15
Doctor: (to proposed purchaser of practice) You have seen the books, the office, and met the staff. The practice is a turnkey operation. You should be able to do very well here. With a little hard work....

Lesson: The words "with a little hard work" should signal that something may be awry that the seller has not been completely honest about. You will need to do your homework to research the practice as thoroughly as possible.

TREATMENT
You may feel an ethical or moral obligation to walk away from any negotiation in which your opponent has been less than candid. Unfortunately, due to the proliferation of this tactic, this is not always a practical alternative. Frequently, the best way to proceed is to not immediately jump to your feet and call your opponent a liar. While this might feel good, it will rarely advance the negotiation process or assist you in achieving your goals. The best way to proceed is to fully prepare by gathering as much negotiation information as possible and, at the crucial juncture, use it as a sledgehammer. This should allow you to seize momentum and power and achieve your goals.

Example 13.16
Proposed purchaser: (to colleague) I know you are looking for $750,000 for your practice. I have checked the books and they look fine. What you failed to tell me is that your HMO status is in serious jeopardy. You just settled your third malpractice suit and a competing practice has been trying to get hospital privileges and move into your area. Normally, I would just walk away from this deal due to your lack of candor. If you really want to sell your practice *today,* give me your bottom-line figure now or your best chance for a sale will be walking out that door in thirty seconds!

Lesson: The doctor has turned his opponent's tactic against him. He has gained power and momentum in the negotiation.

Tactic 5: Outrageous Opening Offer or Demand

DIAGNOSIS

This tactic is usually easy to diagnose. When using this tactic, your opponent takes the advice of "leave yourself room to negotiate" to the extreme and opens the negotiation with a grossly inflated offer or demand.

Example 13.17

Consultant: (to doctor) We can come in and straighten out your billing, accounts receivables, computer software, your hardware, and your leasing arrangements for the flat fee of $100,000. It sounds initially like a lot, but over two to three years it will more than pay for itself.

TREATMENT

You need to recognize the ploy and refuse to play into the hands of the opponent by getting into an auction type of negotiation. Alternatively, a response of a ridiculous counteroffer may jolt your opponent back to reality.

Example 13.18

Doctor: (to consultant) Your opening bid is so high it is ridiculous. Why don't you rethink your position and, when you have something in the ballpark, give me a call?

Lesson: This is the direct defense. If your opponent comes back in the ballpark, you can start negotiations in earnest. If he does not, you will not be wasting any more time negotiating with him.

Example 13.19
Doctor: (to consultant) Your $100,000 figure is ridiculous. We were thinking in terms of $1,000.

Lesson: Another direct defense. She has responded with an equally ridiculous offer. This counteroffer communicates to your opponent the fact that he is far afield and leaves substantial room for future negotiations.

Tactic 6: Belly Up

DIAGNOSIS
This tactic is easy to diagnose. When using this tactic, your opponent puts himself at your mercy and refuses to negotiate. It is a psychological tactic in which your opponents hope to manipulate you to bend over backwards to be fair due to their frank admission of their inability or unwillingness to negotiate.

Example 13.20
Colleague: (to doctor) Fred, you know me. I am a doctor and not a negotiator. Pay me what is fair and let's be done with it.

Example 13.21
Colleague: (to doctor) Fred, you know my family situation. You know I am in no position to negotiate. I have to trust you to be fair. We have always been fair to each other in the past.

TREATMENT

You should not fall for this tactic by giving additional concessions to your opponent because he has gone "belly up." You need to recognize the belly-up tactic for what it is, a psychological ploy to wring additional concessions from a sympathetic doctor. To combat this tactic you need to stick firmly with your fair offer.

Example 13.22

Fred: (to colleague) I try to be fair. I am a doctor also and not a negotiator. What I can offer is…, which is fair to both of us.

Lesson: The doctor turned the situation around by stressing what was fair to *him*. Additional concessions were not given. The doctor had the strength of will to stand firm in the face of his opponent's powerful psychological ploy.

Tactic 7: Anchoring

DIAGNOSIS

This may be the most difficult tactic for the physician negotiator to diagnose. It may be used when your opponent suspects that you do not know, or have not set a price or value on, your service, program, or product. Your opponent knows that if she can throw out a price, you may get psychologically anchored to that price area and fail or be afraid to ask for what the service is really worth. Your opponent also knows that you may be afraid to embarrass yourself by questioning the anchor price.

Example 13.23

TV producer: Doctor, we have a tentative agreement on a five-part series of ten-minute segments on "You and Your Health." We normally pay $100 for short segments, but because you are a physician, we will make it $150. What day next week is good for you to film the segments?

Doctor: I will be losing one to two days out of the office. I need to get at least $1,500 for the five segments.

TV producer: You doctors are tough. Okay. You got the $1,500, but keep it confidential. We don't want the rest of the talent to get jealous.

Lesson: The doctor got anchored to the initial offer and did not even look at what his services might really be worth.

TREATMENT

You need to accept the initial offer as just one piece of information. You should not fixate on it when determining value and asking price. You should not be intimidated by the anchor price and should not be embarrassed to question where the anchor figure comes from. You need to determine your value independently and look at the initial offer as merely the opponent's attempt to get you to stick close to the anchor. Do not let the anchor figure in any way impede your assessment of the true value of your opponent's offer.

Example 13.24

Doctor: To do a professional job, I will have to spend a considerable amount of time writing and researching the scripts. I estimate that each segment will take four

to five hours to script. My normal consulting fee is
$300 an hour, so I will require....
Producer: Doctor, we are not "60 Minutes" here, but
we can probably get you....

Lesson: The doctor simply refused to be anchored.
His demand was based upon his own independent
valuation of his services, not his opponent's opening
offer.

Tactic 8: You Have Got to Do Better than That

DIAGNOSIS

This tactic should be easy to diagnose. Here your
opponent feigns surprise at your initial demand and
requests that you immediately reconsider your position.
What your opponent is really asking for is for you to
bid against yourself. (See page 43 on bidding against
yourself.) Bidding against yourself is one of the biggest
mistakes a physician negotiator can ever make.

Example 13.25

Opponent: (to doctor) Doctor, we have your price of
$25,000 for the consulting contract. Just because we
are a large company does not mean that we throw
money around. You have got to do better than that.

Lesson: The doctor has been asked to bid against
herself. She should not do so.

TREATMENT

You need to recognize this as another psychological
tactic and ploy. Your opponent is trying to intimidate
you into lowering your price by playing on your fears
that you priced yourself out of the market, failed to

consider a crucial factor, or made some other error. What makes this tactic so effective is that your opponent does not specify the mistake you made, but lets your imagination run wild as to all the possible things you could have done wrong. The savvy opponent knows that physicians do not like to make mistakes and will do almost anything to avoid being embarrassed. To combat this tactic you cannot be intimidated and should put the ball back in your opponent's court. Do not bid against yourself!

Example 13.26
Opponent: Doctor, we have your price of $25,000. You have to do better than that.
Doctor: We took great pains to come up with a fair price. What do you have in mind?

Lesson: The doctor is not intimidated nor does she allow herself to be browbeaten into bidding against herself. A counteroffer is demanded from the opponent. The doctor does not bid against herself.

Tactic 9: Pleading Poverty

DIAGNOSIS
You should normally be able to spot this tactic without too much difficulty. The tactic involves your opponents pleading that they only have limited funds to accomplish the job. It is therefore not their fault, or so they argue, that they cannot pay you more. Consider the following example.

Example 13.27
Nonprofit agency executive director: Doctor, we know your time is worth $25,000, but the budget I am working with only has $20,000 allocated.

Lesson: What the opponent is really saying is that some third party/agency has made a mistake in setting its budget unrealistically low and, as a result, you should pay for its mistake.

TREATMENT
You need to recognize that the party who makes a mistake normally should pay for the mistake. You also need to understand that many opponents intentionally come to the table with their "hands tied" as a ploy to strengthen their bargaining positions. To combat this tactic you need to turn the focus of the negotiation back to what you require. You will need to justify your demands to make them more effective. You can also point out to your opponents ways in which they can free up more money.

Example 13.28
Nonprofit agency executive director: Doctor, we know your time is worth $25,000, but the budget I am working with only has $20,000 allocated.
Doctor: I appreciate your position, but budgets are not engraved in stone. See if you can get yours corrected to reflect my true value so we can proceed with the project.

Lesson: The doctor correctly refused to accept her opponent's claims of poverty. She suggested to her opponent ways to make more money available and focused the negotiation on her true value.

Tactic 10: Limited Authority

DIAGNOSIS

Diagnosing this tactic requires you to determine the level of authority that your opponent has. (See pages 39-48 on authority.) The best way to do this is to ask early in the negotiation.

Example 13.29

Doctor: (to executive) As I understand it, you have no final authority to negotiate today. You are on a fact-finding mission.

TREATMENT

You need to insist on the opponent producing someone with the authority to negotiate. You should refuse to negotiate until this occurs.

Example 13.30

Doctor: (to executive) I understand that you are only authorized to obtain my demands and pass them along to management. Before we start to negotiate, we need to get someone in here with the authority to finalize the terms of the agreement.

Lesson: The physician has acted correctly in refusing to negotiate with the person with limited authority. She has correctly demanded that she deal with someone in authority before she will begin to negotiate.

Additional Tactics

You may be exposed to other negotiation tactics as well. Following is a list of such tactics, the offensive statements, and brief defensive replies.

The nibble
Offense: "If you throw in the service, I will buy the system."
Defense: "I am sorry, I don't have the authority to do that. You can see the price list on the wall."

False flattery: You're the best!
Offense: "We know you are the best physician for the assignment...."
Defense: "I appreciate the flattery, but I can't pay college tuition with kind words and thoughts."

The screamer
Offense: (screaming) "I need an answer **NOW!**"
Defense: (softly) "I hear that you may be upset. Maybe we should lower our voices so we can hear each other better."

Need to talk it over
Offense: "I would love to agree today, but I need to talk to my partner."
Defense: "Call him or her now and let's go over it. You can use my phone."

Trial balloon: Would you be willing to accept...?
Offense: "Would you be willing to accept $150,000 for the position as outlined?"
Defense: "Are you offering $150,000?"

The staller
Offense: "I need more time to think it over."

Defense: "Are two days ok? How about one week?"

Brinksmanship
Offense: "Well, we still have three days to the drop-dead deadline."
Defense: "We know the deadline. We don't know if last minute negotiations will work here."

Bids
Offense: "We are putting this out to bid and then will be interviewing the lowest bidder."
Defense: "We will bid, but we would like you to call us last and give us an opportunity to match any other bids."

Team player
Offense: "Our offer is $125,000. Be a team player and accept it."
Defense: "You would not want an unhappy team member. I need $150,000."

Think of the future
Offense: "We are offering you $95,000 for year one, but as you get more experience, we will take care of you."
Defense: "I need taking care of now—$125,000." *(or)* "Let's put in writing the salary for each subsequent year."

Limited time offer
Offense: "This offer is only good for 24 hours."
Defense: "If you really want me, I am sure you will give me the weekend to think this over and talk to my spouse."

Selection from a limited menu

Offense: "You deserve $120,000. All I can offer is between $100,000 and $110,000."

Defense: "I will take what I deserve…$120,000."

Renogotiation

Offense: "I need $160,000, not the $150,000 we agreed to yesterday."

Defense: "I cannot negotiate under these conditions. We do not renegotiate terms already agreed to."

Chapter 14 Team Negotiating

You will often be forced to negotiate as part of or against a team or committee. Such negotiations require special techniques. These techniques are discussed in the following sections.

Size and Composition of the Team

The size of the negotiating team is important. When selecting the size of the team, you should consider the size of the opposing team, what each proposed team member has to offer, and the amount of time available to negotiate. To avoid being worn down by the opposing team, your team should be approximately the same size as that of the opponent. Each proposed team member should be evaluated on their ability to help prepare, their specific area of expertise, and their ability to get along with fellow team members. Leaving a person off the team who will later have to approve the proposed deal may make it more difficult to obtain their approval for a deal they have not personally negotiated. The larger the team, the longer the negotiation is likely to take. When your opposition has tighter time constraints than you have, you can capitalize on this by producing a large negotiating team.

Selection of the physician negotiation team leader is a crucial decision. It should not be taken lightly. The physician selected should be the most skilled and experienced negotiator and a physician who is well respected by all the team members. Generally, physicians who are self-confident, flexible, and exercise good business judgment make good team leaders.

Example 14.1

Doctor: (to proposed team members) The "opposition" has four team members and so we will go with four ourselves. We need someone to pull together the history of past negotiations and to research the salary structure of other similar groups, a team leader, a number cruncher, and a listener. What are your recommendations? Let's remember they are the ones that need to get a deal quickly.

Lesson: The doctor is thinking of how to compose the team. Team members should be given duties that correspond to their strengths. The researchers should research, the listeners should listen, and the leader should negotiate. If they want to put additional pressure on the other side, they may want to increase the size of their negotiation team. This will slow down the process, which may be helpful in gaining concessions.

Controlling the Information Flow

It is essential to tightly control the flow of information coming from any and all team members. Ideally, the team leader should also act as the sole spokesperson. This will avoid leaks of confidential information or contradictory statements. To combat this problem, information that is not to be revealed should be discussed and agreed to in advance of the negotiation. All team members must be made to understand that even the most innocent sounding question could be an attempt by an opponent to find out confidential information. When properly prepared and coached, the team members will tightly control the information flow. (See pages 39-82 on getting as much information and revealing as little information as possible.)

Example 14.2

Negotiation team member What time is your flight out of here tonight?

Opposing team member: We are all catching the last flight at 7:00 P.M.

Lesson: The opposing team now has better information as to the time constraints of the team. Information has been disseminated. A better answer may have been, "I'm not sure, Doctor [team leader] is in charge of those arrangements."

Example 14.3

Negotiation team member: What's with Dr. Dunlop? Why is she being so difficult?

Opposing team member: She is under a lot of pressure to get this deal done today.

Lesson: Harmful information has been revealed.

Example 14.4

Negotiation team member: What time is your flight out of here tonight?

Opposing team member: Why do you think we will finish tonight?

Lesson: A request for information has been cleverly reversed into a request for information from the other team.

Example 14.5
Negotiation team member: What's with Dr. Dunlop?
Why is she being so difficult?
Opposing team member: I don't know. Why don't
you go back and ask her?

Lesson: The team player has correctly refused to give
out the requested information. Had he done so, he may
have revealed critical information concerning the
team's pressures, needs, and desires.

Goal Setting

The first and most crucial negotiation is the one
amongst the team members when they set and agree
upon their goals. The team leader should help ensure
that the goals are practical, understood, and most
importantly, agreed upon by *all* the team members.
(See pages 120-122 on setting goals.) A unified front is
needed to negotiate effectively.

Consensus building is crucial to the smooth
running of a negotiation team. When a team member is
unhappy about the negotiation's goals, she should be
convinced or asked to leave the team. Nothing can be
more damaging to a negotiating team than an unhappy
physician who snipes at other team members and whose
real goal is to prove them wrong. Team leaders need to
get their team members to sign off on as many crucial
decisions as possible *before* the negotiation process
begins.

During the negotiation itself, the team will have
to stay flexible (see pages 112-113 on flexibility). They
may need to caucus frequently to redefine their goals.
Team members should buy into this process before the
negotiation begins, set their goals high, and leave

themselves adequate room to negotiate. (See page 139 on adequate room to negotiate.)

Example 14.6
Doctor: (to colleagues) We have agreement for our bottom line on the length of the proposed contract, the geographic area covered, and the number of physicians required. The last item we need to agree on is cost. Nancy, I understand you feel strongly on this issue. Convince us....

Lesson: The team members either all need to agree or Nancy needs to be left off the team. Her presence on a team where she is negotiating something she does not believe in could be extremely detrimental.

<u>Signaling</u>

You need to anticipate the need to signal each other at key junctures during the negotiation. You should have prearranged signals for getting a team member to stop talking, notifying each other when an opponent is intentionally or unintentionally misstating the truth, and communicating that the team members need to caucus to discuss a change in strategy or make a key concession.

Be cautious not to inadvertently tip off your opponents that you need to talk or caucus. If you ask for a break/caucus as soon as an issue is brought up or comes to a head, this is a clear signal that you are concerned and are at least considering a compromise or concession. When you do ask for a break, you should have an excuse for this requested break prepared.

Example 14.7
Doctor: (to fellow team member, lightly) Fred, thank you for all of that information. Let's let Andy take the lead for a moment.

Lesson: What is being said here is, "Fred, shut your big mouth! Andy, please try to clean up this mess." This is much better than saying, "Fred, enough. I didn't want you to tell them that."

Example 14.8
Doctor: (to fellow team member and opposition) We must be mistaken, then. I thought our research showed....

Lesson: This is a clever way to correct a wrong answer given by a team member. It should be used as a signal to say, "Be careful when discussing this area, we need to talk."

Example 14.9
Doctor: (to opponent and team members) I need to take a break. We old guys need to get up and stretch every few hours.

Lesson: A good excuse to have a break. A bad excuse would have been, "Let's take a break. Your offer is very tempting and I want to discuss it with my team members."

Example 14.10
Opponent: (to doctors during team negotiation) We need full coverage seven days a week at the emergency

room. We know you offered four days, but what we need is seven days.

Doctor: We need to take a break right about now.

Lesson: This is a bad way to take a needed break. What you are signaling here to your opponent is that since you want to discuss it immediately, seven days may in fact be acceptable.

Example 14.11

Opponent: We need full coverage seven days a week.

Doctor: We need a lot of things also. How about more money, increased staff...?

Opponent: If you want to talk money, we can now.

Five minutes later...

Doctor: I need to take a break. We old guys need to get up and stretch every few hours. Let's take ten. Okay?

Lesson: The team will talk about the coverage issue during the break, but this point was well disguised by the doctor.

Taking Notes

You should assign one or more team members to take notes during the negotiation and to listen actively. This team member should be a good listener (see pages 64-82 on active listening skills) and should note not only what is being agreed to, but also the concerns expressed, important gestures, dissension in the ranks of the opponent, and other nonverbal cues. (See pages 71-74 on nonverbal communication.) These notes can be very helpful during team caucuses.

All notes, deadlines, messages, etc. should be taken by the team members and not left lying on the negotiation table during breaks. You can assume that your opposition will most likely read notes left in plain view. Some negotiators specialize in reading upside down, so caution should be exercised even if your opponent is sitting on the opposite side of the negotiation table.

Example 14.12

Doctor: (during caucus, reading from notes) Each time we talked about money, Jeff (opponent) would sit back in his chair and fold his arms. He would then whisper to Becky (opponent). It was Tom who seemed to be the most sympathetic. At one point he was starting to say we had a point but was cut off by Jeff. Leslie (opponent) agreed with almost everything Tom had to say. It seems to me that Tom is the key here. He is our best hope of getting a fair price.

Lesson: The note taker was able to make these detailed observations because his *only* role in the negotiations was active listening and note taking. The note taker is one of the most important members of the team. A good note taker is like a good offensive lineman in football. That person must be able to accept the fact that even though he is more important to success, the quarterback often gets 98% of the glory.

Caucusing

You should caucus as frequently and for as long as necessary to modify the team's goals and strategy. Caucusing may also be necessary to maintain a consensus and goodwill amongst the team members.

The comments of opposing team members should not deter you from caucusing as often as necessary. An added benefit of frequent caucuses is that such frequent meetings tend to disguise the fact that a caucus is being held because of some recently discussed issue.

During the break, it is essential to hear from all team members who have something constructive to say. The physician team leader will have to maintain tight control over the team during these short breaks in order to make the best use of the time available. You will need to maintain security and not permit your team meeting to be overheard by the opposing team.

Example 14.13
Doctor: We will be taking a fifteen- to twenty-minute break to talk things over amongst ourselves.
Opponent: Another break? I think that is the fourth one already and we are not even finished with half of the issues. You guys need to get your act together.
Doctor: Why don't you use these few minutes to sharpen your proposal instead of complaining? Whining is not really consistent with your tough guy image.

Lesson: The doctor is not intimidated by his opponent's comments. He takes the break regardless and gains power by responding strongly to his opponent's negative comments.

Example 14.14
Physician team leader: (to team) Okay. We have twenty minutes. Let's spend ten minutes going around the room brainstorming and leave ourselves ten minutes

to come up with our three best alternatives. Joanne, why don't you start? Fred, keep an eye on the time.

Lesson: The team leader keeps tight control on the meeting in order to assure that no time is wasted. The goal of three best alternatives is set down before the negotiation recommences.

Example 14.15
Doctor: (to team members) Do you hear the yelling and shouting coming out of their caucus room? I guess they are not all on the same page. We might be able to exploit this divisiveness.

Lesson: Make sure that the other side cannot hear what is being said in your caucus. If they can, you could be giving up highly damaging and highly confidential material.

Resolving Team Disagreements

You should anticipate that disagreements will arise amongst team members. You should set up an agreed-upon method for resolving these disputes *before* the negotiation begins. Getting the team members to buy into the method for resolving internal disputes will help reduce the chances that a team member will become unhappy, uncooperative, or destructive. If the team has to check with a higher authority, the team leader should make the call herself on a secure line. The team should disguise and not reveal to the opposition the specific issue(s) under discussion. Such revelations can undercut the apparent authority and power of the team and its leader.

Example 14.16

Team leader: (to team members) We agree, then, that if anyone has a problem with the way the negotiation is going, he or she will signal me. I will take a break. At the break, we will agree amongst ourselves on how to proceed. In the event that we cannot agree and we are deadlocked, I will cast the deciding vote. Are we all okay with this method?

Lesson: A method to resolve internal disputes is critically important. A divided front during team negotiations can be fatal.

Team Negotiation Tactics

The two most commonly used team negotiation tactics should be discussed by your team in advance. These techniques are "divide and conquer" and the "weak link." Team members need to be able to quickly identify these tactics for what they are and should respond appropriately.

DIVIDE AND CONQUER

Divide and conquer involves your opponent trying to drive a wedge into the physician negotiation team. The hope is that this wedge will lead to squabbling. The hoped for result is the team losing its focus and being substantially weakened. A wedge remark should be directly responded to by the person it was targeted toward. This will help display the most unified front possible.

Example 14.17
Group practice leader: (to team of ten physicians being bought out) We have offered you $20 million. You have ten partners. That works out to $2 million each.
(Looking at the youngest partner) How much more than $2 million each do you need? That is, of course, based on the assumption that each of you will be getting 10%. Since your income production was more or less equal, we just assumed that you would each get an equal share.

Lesson: The opponent's wedge is used in an attempt to get the doctors' team fighting about money amongst themselves. This would naturally lead to disunity.

Example 14.18
Group practice leader: (to team of ten physicians) We have offered you $20 million. Each of you would get an equal share.
Young partner: Put your wedge back in your bag. This negotiation would be close to being completed if you offered us a reasonable amount.

Lesson: The target of the wedge attacked it head on. The team has stopped the wedge and gained power by showing its strength of unity.

WEAK LINK

In the "weak link" tactic, your opponent will quickly identify your physician team member who is most ill-suited to be a negotiator. If a physician team member is unduly concerned about being well liked or is inexperienced or unduly afraid of deadlock, then he is susceptible to becoming the weak link. A sports analogy is helpful in explaining the weak link tactic. In basketball and football, the offense quickly identifies the weakest defender, isolates that person, and then takes advantage of the defender's shortcomings. The same tactics are used during team negotiations.

When you become aware of a weak link on your negotiating team, you should get that person off the team as quickly as possible. If this is not a practical solution, sit next to the weak link and do not let him or her out of your sight for even one minute. The weak link is particularly vulnerable in ongoing negotiations that are spread out over days or weeks. One well-placed phone call to the weak link by a savvy opponent can result in serious information leaks, major concessions, and fatal damage to the negotiation. Leave the weak link back in the office as far away as possible from the negotiation site.

Example 14.19
Team opponent: (to doctor during break) Joe, can you help me carry the box of printouts?

When Joe is isolated from the team...
Joe, I am telling you this as a friend. Nothing against your team and team leader, but they are ruining *your* career and future in medicine. You have a reputation of twenty years of excellence, integrity, honesty, and now to throw it all away over these issues that have nothing to do with you. Other doctors have been talking. Don't let your team push you around. Remember, after all is said and done, it is *your* reputation.

Lesson: Joe should have been left back at the office. Failing this, he should not have been allowed to be alone with an opponent. The team leader should have "double-teamed" the opponent and sent another team member to escort the weak link.

Agendas

You need to deal effectively with any disparate agendas that physicians may have prior to, or which could develop during, the negotiation. Team members may be trying to impress the opposition, line up future consulting work or employment, and build up goodwill for future use. Each of these individual agendas can be damaging to the team as a whole. This problem is particularly troublesome if the team members are not co-employees or partners, but are instead independent contractors brought together with the express purpose of negotiating an agreement for their mutual benefit. The apparent and hidden agendas of the physician team members need to be addressed and reined in by the team leader and the team prior to and during the negotiation.

Example 14.20
Doctors on the same team to their opponents...
Doctor Washington: We are looking at developing a protocol. We would recommend a needs assessment, development of hard data, and interpreting the data. This consulting work should be done before we develop educational programs. We are looking at three to six months of consulting work. As you know, this is my area of specialty.
Doctor Lopez: While I agree with Joe that the data is important, I think we can proceed immediately to develop the distance learning programs and seminars. As you know, this is *my* area of specialty.

Lesson: Team members need to be team players. If they are not, they should not be on the team. If this situation occurs during an ongoing negotiation, the team leader should find an excuse to take a break and then take firm control of the situation.

Flexibility

Your team needs to remain flexible. The more rigid the team becomes, the less open it is to reason, compromise, and concessions. (See pages 112-113 on flexibility.) It is the responsibility of the team leader to remind the team periodically that just because they all agree on a point does not make it a fact and does not mean they cannot and should not remain flexible.

Example 14.21
Physician team leader: (to team) We all agree $3 million, not a penny less. Our practice is worth every penny. We all have worked too long and hard to sell ourselves short. We will hang tough, but we may need to rethink our goals if we can't get the $3 million.

Lesson: The team leader reinforces the unity of the team with the $3 million demand. He also, however, prepares them to be flexible if that goal appears to be unattainable.

Chapter 15 Negotiating for the Retention of an Attorney

Retaining counsel or a law firm can be a traumatic and very costly experience. Unfortunately, it is very likely that you will need to hire an attorney many times over the course of your career. What you pay for her legal services are 100% negotiable. In order to successfully negotiate with attorneys regarding retention, you will need to understand law office economics, the legal fee arrangements that are available, the best arrangements, when the best time is to hire an attorney, how to get better fee agreements by being a good client, and the criteria to use in selecting counsel.

Law Office Economics

You will be able to reduce legal costs through a better understanding of law office economics. This understanding needs to be applied with the use of selected negotiating techniques. Most law offices are set up with the partners running the firm and obtaining new business. The routine, time-consuming work is then referred to less experienced associates. These associates are then "billed out" at a multiple of their salaries. The client pays a very high hourly rate for the partners, lower rates to train the associates, and as much of the expenses of running the law firm as the firm can get away with. **You must also keep in mind that there is no limit to the amount of legal work that can be done on even a routine matter, if an attorney knows that she will be paid for it.** The first rule in negotiating with an attorney is, therefore, to be very careful to not give the attorney a blank check. Consider the following examples.

Example 15.1

Law firm partner: Doctor, I understand the issue. The legal question is the validity of the covenant not to compete that you signed two years ago as a young, inexperienced physician. We will look at the corporate practice of medicine doctrine, anti-trust, and any other theory that we can come up with to invalidate your five-year covenant. We will need a $5,000 retainer and will apply that against our billing rate of $290 an hour plus expenses....

Doctor: Fine. I need to get out from under that covenant.... It is stopping me from taking advantage of a wonderful opportunity.

Doctor leaves office.

Partner: (to associate, who is being paid $50 an hour, as he tosses the file on her desk) Nancy, I need you to research this covenant not to compete. I want you to do a thorough job. I will need a detailed memorandum. The client will be coming in on Friday and I will need it before then. Take a look at the *Berlin v. Sarah Bush Lincoln Center* case at 664 N.E.2d 337 (1996) and *Holden v. Rockford Memorial Hospital* 678 N.E.2d 342 (1997). They might help. Any questions?

Associate: Is there any limit on time or expenses here?

Partner: (laughing) We are dealing with a doctor who has agreed to pay the firm $290 an hour plus expenses.

Associate: Got it. You will have the memo on Thursday even if I have to work on it day and night until then.

Partner: I am glad we understand each other.

Lesson: The unsophisticated doctor has, in effect, given the law firm a blank check. He will be paying $290 an hour for work done almost exclusively by a new associate who is paid $50 an hour by the firm. The doctor has put no restrictions on the type of expenses, their cost, or their mark up. As difficult as it may be to believe, the majority of doctors who retain lawyers and law firms "negotiate" in the same way and achieve the same results as the doctor in this example.

Example 15.2

Law firm partner: Doctor, I understand the issue. The legal question is the validity of the covenant not to compete…$5,000 retainer…billing rate of $290 an hour plus expenses….

Doctor: Before we discuss fees, have you had much experience in these covenant not to compete cases?

Partner: Yes. I have handled three or four cases like this in the past two years alone.

Doctor: I take it you will not be billing me for original research if you already have many of the issues briefed.

Partner: Well, each case is unique…. They depend upon the facts…. But, obviously we will not bill you for work previously done.

Doctor: Will an associate be doing the research?

Partner: Yes, but I will be reviewing the work and giving you my opinion. That is what you are *really* paying for.

Doctor: Do you want to charge me a reduced rate for the associate's time or would a blended rate of $175 an hour work better for you?

Partner: (reluctantly) We can go with the blended rate of $175.

Doctor: As this is a routine research project, the only expenses should be the actual Westlaw charges and fax and copying costs, correct?

Partner: Yes. We will bill you those at our own cost.

Doctor: I would hope that this would not take more than ten hours of work. Would a $1,750 retainer be reasonable...?

Partner: (anticipating the next request) Yes...and I will call you before we exceed your retainer.

Doctor: Thank you.

Partner: (to associate, throwing the file on her desk) Nancy, I need you to research this covenant not to compete and do a memo for Thursday. Pull out the memo in the *Jones* case and *Kahn* case. The issues are basically the same and look at the *Berlin* and *Holden* cases. Keep the bill under $1,750. No cell phone calls, overtime for staff, meals, or taxi rides. This doctor will not stand for that stuff....

Associate: One lean and mean memo...no fat, no frills, no extras.

Partner: I am glad we understand each other.

Lesson: The doctor did not give the attorney a blank check. He verified that the work would not be time consuming, that he would be billed a blended rate, that there would be no extravagant expenses, and that he would be notified immediately if his retainer was exceeded.

Legal Fee Arrangements

You need to understand the various legal fee arrangements that are available. You should strive to obtain the fee arrangement that reduces your exposure to legal costs while at the same time maintaining or increasing the attorney's incentive to successfully conclude the case. The legal fee arrangements that are generally available and their uses are described in Box 15.1. The best fee arrangement for you to negotiate will depend upon the type of case that you have and the type of lawyer that you need.

Box 15.1

Types of Attorney's Fee Arrangements

1. Contingent fee: Your attorney will receive a percentage of your recovery (i.e., 33⅓% in personal injury matters). This method can also be used in contractual and some other types of disputes.
2. Fixed fee: Your attorney will receive a flat fee for representing you in a case (i.e., $2,500 for a minor criminal case).
3. Hourly fee and expenses: In complex matters your attorney will charge you his or her hourly billing rate plus expenses (i.e., $250 per hour and expenses).
4. Blended fee and expenses: The attorney will charge you a combination of the associates' and partners' billing rates plus expenses.
5. Reverse contingency fee: You and the attorney agree on a worst-case scenario and you agree to pay the attorney a percentage of anything he or she can save you from that amount.

CONTINGENCY FEE

When you are the plaintiff in a personal injury case or involved in a speculative case, you are normally better off seeking a contingency fee arrangement. There are three main advantages to this type of fee arrangement. First, you will typically not have to pay any up-front retainers, fees, or expenses to initiate the litigation. Second, if you lose the case, you will not be obligated to pay any legal fee. (Note, however, that most contingent fee agreements do provide that you will be responsible for the attorney's expenses.) Third, and most importantly, the attorney representing you has a substantial and significant financial incentive to win the case. If the attorney loses, she gets nothing. If the attorney wins, she gets 33% of the award or whatever the contingency fee is that you negotiated. An example of a speculative case where you should attempt to get a contingency fee arrangement would be suing for lost profits in a medical practice. By requesting a contingency fee arrangement, you can quickly determine the viability of your claim. If one or more attorneys turn you down and insist on being paid by the hour, you should think long and hard before investing your time and money in hourly representation for the claim.

On contingency cases, you will frequently be presented with a standard form calling for a 30% or 33% legal fee. This fee is *always* negotiable. Because less than 5% of cases ever go to trial, one good tactic is to insist on a fee reduction if the case is settled before trial. You should also remember that, when hiring an attorney on a contingency fee, you should hire the best attorney that you can find.

Example 15.3
Doctor: (to attorney, showing him the documents) We would like to sue a former partner for breaching his contract, stealing patients, and for the profits our practice lost.
Attorney: (looking over documents) This looks like a solid case. We would be pleased to represent you. We will stand a good chance of winning.

Doctor: We would like you to represent us on a contingency basis....
Attorney: No can do. These cases are too speculative...there are too many variables.

Lesson: By insisting on a contingent fee agreement, the doctor has determined what the attorney really thinks about this case. If two or three other attorneys also refuse to accept such an arrangement, the doctor should strongly consider not pursuing the case.

Example 15.4
Attorney: Doctor, here is our standard preprinted contingency calling for a 33% legal fee. Please read it and sign it.
Doctor: I would like to make one change. I need the 33% reduced to 25% if this case is settled prior to trial.
Attorney: Well, doctor, we do not normally reduce....
Doctor: (cutting him off) As you know, there are 7,500 certified trial specialists in this state. I am sure that when I call two or three....
Attorney: Give me a few minutes to make that change.

Lesson: The amount of the fee is *always* negotiable. This is especially true if you have a good case.

Example 15.5
When Pennzoil sued Texaco, it hired nationally known trial attorney Joe Jamail on a contingency basis. He obtained one of the largest judgments of our time, $10.53 billion. His legal fee has been estimated at $350 to $500 million. They were happy to pay the fee because they knew that without Attorney Jamail, there would have been no $10.53 billion verdict.

Lesson: It is in your interest when prosecuting a contingency fee case to hire the best attorney that you can.

FIXED FEE

There are advantages and disadvantages to fixed fee arrangements. The chief benefit is that you know the cost of your representation and can budget accordingly. You need to understand the substantial drawbacks to this arrangement as well. The three chief drawbacks are, first, that the fee may be set too high to take into account things that might go wrong. Second, if the fee is too low, the attorney may lose interest in your case. Third, counsel may have a less experienced associate handle the case. Consider the following examples.

Example 15.6
Doctor: You charged me $5,000 for this contract problem and you resolved it with one fifteen-minute phone call.
Attorney: It took me twenty years of experience to learn who to call and what to say.

Lesson: A fixed fee may result in overpaying for legal services.[1]

Example 15.7
Doctor: I have left twelve messages. You never return my calls.
Attorney: There is only so much time I can devote to this case due to our fee arrangement. I am doing the best I can.

---

[1] In this case, $20,000 per hour.

Lesson: The attorney losing interest is a serious risk when the arrangement is for a fixed fee.

Example 15.8
Doctor: (to new associate in court) Who are you? Where is Attorney Relief?
Associate: He was tied up with another matter. Don't worry, I have been doing most of the work on your case anyway.

Lesson: If the fee is fixed, you may end up with an inexperienced attorney doing the actual work.

HOURLY FEE

The successful physician negotiator understands that in most cases in which he or she retains counsel, a request will be made for payment of an hourly fee plus expenses. The hourly fee could range from $125 to $350 an hour or more. The expenses can range from photocopying charges to airfare, hotels, cabs, meals, etc. A complex case in which the physician is paying by the hour can be a financially draining experience. The savvy physician negotiator knows ten ways to help reduce this exposure.

1. Ask for a reduced hourly rate

Example 15.9
Doctor: I understand you normally charge $350 an hour. I normally pay $150 an hour. Can we split the difference (see pages 177-179 on splitting the difference) and agree on $250 an hour?
Attorney: Okay.

Lesson: The hourly rate is always negotiable. Note, however, that when attorneys reduce their rates, they can make up for it by billing more hours.

2. Ask for a reduced rate for associates' time and travel

Example 15.10
Doctor: (to attorney) I don't mind paying for associates' time and for travel, but can we agree to $150 an hour for associates' time and 50% for travel time if any is needed?

Lesson: If you don't ask for concessions, you will never get any.

3. Get an estimate of total cost

Example 15.11
Doctor: Can you give me an estimate/ballpark figure on what you anticipate the total cost of this case will be? (See pages 183-186 on estimates.)
Attorney: It will all depend on how cooperative the other side will be. A rough estimate is between....

Lesson: It will be difficult for the attorney to later exceed this estimate. The doctor has given herself some protection.

4. Request billing by the tenth of the hour

Example 15.12
Doctor: (to attorney) In light of your hourly rate, I would prefer to get billed by the tenth of the hour and not by the quarter of an hour. This would be fairer to

me and will more accurately reflect the time actually spent.

Lesson: This is a good argument and is difficult for the attorney to refute.

5. Set a maximum fee not to be exceeded

Example 15.13
Doctor: Your fee is $250 an hour with a maximum of $15,000, correct?
Attorney: Yes, and we will do our best to resolve this case quickly.

Lesson: The savvy physician has capped his legal fee exposure.

6. Ask for reduced charges for standard forms and agreements

Example 15.14
Doctor: This is boilerplate stuff, all you'll need to do is change your form. The time required will be minimal.
Attorney: It will require some modification.

Lesson: The doctor has lowered the fee expectations of the attorney.

7. Request weekly or monthly itemized billing

Example 15.15
Doctor: I will need monthly itemized billing.

Lesson: This helps the client monitor the legal costs. Additionally, she knows exactly how the attorneys' time is being spent (e.g., 14 hours on inter-office conferences)

8. Request efficient handling of the case ("Ask or ye may not receive")

Example 15.16
Doctor: I am not the tobacco industry with unlimited resources. Do a good, thorough job, but no excesses.

Lesson: The attorney is put on notice that the legal bill will be scrutinized.

9. Request reduced billing for attorney conferences and for file reviews

Example 15.17
Doctor: I don't want to be getting any bills for lengthy conferences or file reviews.

Lesson: The doctor has taken away some billing ammunition from the attorney.

10. Strive to resolve the case by settlement or alternative dispute resolution before incurring large legal bills

Example 15.18
Doctor: I want you to make an offer to settle this now, before we go through all those costly motions and discovery.

Lesson: The doctor points out to the attorney he is interested in a quick, fair, inexpensive resolution.

Expenses

Many law firms substantially mark up their expenses and view them as an excellent additional source of revenue. You need to put strict limits on traditional law firm expenses, such as photocopies, airline and other travel, copying, cellular phone calls, overtime for paralegals and secretaries, hotel bills, meals, cabs, and limousines. You should demand itemized receipts for all expenses. You should also demand the apportionment of expenses if two or more cases/projects are being done at the same time at the same location.

Example 15.19

Doctor: We have an agreement on your hourly rate. I am very concerned about the possibility of out of control expenses....

Attorney: I can assure you....

Doctor: That's what I am looking for...you to be personally responsible for keeping a sharp eye on expenses incurred and billed. What we both want to avoid is "utilization review" by a legal fee auditing company.

Attorney: What are you looking for specifically?

Doctor: No mark up on faxes, photocopies, or phone calls, no travel or other expenses over $500 without my prior written approval. No eating at five-star restaurants on the road. No first-class airfares, taxi rides, or limo rides without your written approval, overtime charges, hotel bills that contain extra charges for bar bills, x-rated movies, hair cuts, massages...excessive use of cellular phones. We would prefer that large research projects be referred to legal research companies. In other words, please treat my money as carefully as I do.

Attorney: We will do our best.

Doctor: Please prepare an addendum to my fee agreement reflecting our understanding and circulate it to the attorneys who will be working the case.

Lesson: Attorneys can and will bill you for any and all expenses they can get away with. You need to be proactive to prevent yourself from being abused by that practice.

When to Hire an Attorney

The best time to look for, interview, choose, and negotiate with counsel is when you are not desperately in need of services. As in all negotiations, the greater your need for counsel, the less negotiation power you will have. (See pages 83-102 on the best time to negotiate.) Keep in mind that there is a gross excess of attorneys in this country. You should, therefore, always have the power of alternative representation on your side.

Example 15.20

Doctor: (to attorney, handing him a large package of legal materials) We would like you to represent us in this lawsuit. As you can see, we have a hearing on a preliminary injunction in two days. The answer is due.... How much will your fee be?

Attorney: $290 an hour plus expenses.... We will need a retainer of.....

Lesson: If the doctor did not wait until the last minute, he could have shopped around. His delay has left him with few alternatives and very little power in the negotiation.

Example 15.21
Doctor: You don't know me, but I am a cardiologist. I am calling from the Hingham police station. I was picked up a few hours ago for DUI. What I am looking for is for you to come down to the station house, arrange bail, and represent me in the case. This kind of case could destroy my reputation. My husband will be very upset.
Attorney: I will be down to the station house in thirty minutes. Don't say anything to anyone. Have your husband come down to the station with your checkbook. We will discuss my fee when I get there.
Doctor: Thank you.

Lesson: The doctor still has power, even in this situation. If the attorney wants to charge too high of a fee, she can fire her and retain new counsel after she is bailed out. The desperation evident in the doctor's situation has given the attorney additional power in the negotiation.

How to Be a Good Client and Make It Pay Off

One of the most significant concessions you as a potential client can make is the promise to be a good client. This promise can cost you little or nothing, but will be very valuable to your attorney. The qualifications that make a client a good client are listed in Box 15.2. You need to also always keep in mind that the best client for an attorney to have is one that will be coming back to that attorney for significant work in the future. Remember that when an attorney has a difficult client, he may frequently (consciously or subconsciously) charge this client more than the good client.

Box 15.2

The Ten Commandments of Being a Good Client

1. Promptly pay your bills; a physician client who brings in a check when he or she receives a bill is by *definition* a good client.
2. Have your story organized in a chronological fashion, typed neatly.
3. Have all supporting documents available and organized.
4. Make the names, addresses, phone numbers, fax numbers, and e-mail addresses of all witnesses available to counsel.
5. Do not hide "bad" information or mislead counsel.
6. Do not wait until the last second to retain counsel so everything is done in a crisis atmosphere. If counsel has to drop everything to handle your case, it will cost you.
7. Do not continually call the attorney for progress reports. (Ask how often to check in.)
8. Be available. (Don't disappear without leaving contact numbers.)
9. Ask counsel how you can help and then follow this advice.
10. Mention additional work and refer clients. You will get VIP treatment and the best possible hourly rate once you become a significant source of additional legal work for your attorney.

Example 15.22

Doctor: Before we talk about fees, I want to let you know that I will be an excellent client. Noncompliance is a big problem for us and this has made me extremely sensitive to the need to cooperate fully. I also hope to refer substantial amounts of new business to your firm. As you may know, I am president-elect of....

Attorney: We normally bill at $290 an hour. How about a $250 an hour excellent client rate?

Lesson: The promise of possible additional future work is a very powerful negotiating tool. With it, the doctor may turn a competitive negotiation into a cooperative negotiation.

Selection of Counsel

Cost is only one of the criteria for selection of counsel. You should also research and consider the attorney's experience in the specific legal area and whether he or she is too busy. Reputation is important and references should be checked. Finally, make sure that the attorney you retain will be your attorney. You do not want your case handled and managed by an inexperienced attorney in the firm. Always remember that there are a lot of attorneys out there. You can and should shop around.

Example 15.23

Doctor: (to attorney) Your firm has come highly recommended. We are looking for a firm that has significant experience in this area. Will you send me a note with the names and docket numbers of your trials in this area for the past five years and their outcomes? We will need your assurance that you personally will take the key depositions and be lead counsel for any significant motions and the trial. I will need to see a draft sample fee agreement. Use your tightest language for the expenses please and give me the names of five references I can call. I know this is a lot of work, but we are trying to avoid the "beauty contest route."

Lesson: You need to be firm when dealing with attorneys. Do not be afraid to ask pointed questions. Attorneys ask such questions themselves all the time.

Chapter 16 Negotiating Employment, Managed Care, and Other Formal Written Contracts

Many of your most important negotiations will involve formal written contracts. Such negotiations could include employment, managed care, and purchase and sale contracts. An in-depth discussion of the issues and subtleties of negotiating each of these types of contracts is beyond the scope of this book. Indeed, to adequately cover those specific issues would require a series of books. This chapter is designed to assist you with general principles you can apply to *all* negotiations that involve formal written contracts.

Contract Law

You are probably not a lawyer. Reading this next section will not make you a lawyer. However, at a minimum, you will need to have a basic understanding of contract law in order to properly negotiate formal written contracts. More importantly, you need to appreciate and recognize the need to retain and involve a lawyer during many negotiations that involve formal written contracts.

STATE SPECIFIC

The law of contracts is state specific; that is, it varies from state to state. Generally speaking, contract law is founded in the common law, which is precedent from previously decided cases. This common law is modified by statutes passed by the various state legislatures.

INTERPRETATION

If a contract dispute regarding a formal written contract results in litigation, a key issue will be how the written terms of the contract should be interpreted. The key to contract disputes and negotiation, therefore, is precisely which words and terms are in the written contract. A good lawyer plans for contingencies and drafts as tight of language as is possible to protect his client. This planning for contingencies and tightening of language is a major part of contract negotiation. It is also important to realize what a contract does not say and to add appropriate language where needed.

DAMAGES

The law of how to calculate contract damages is too complex to discuss in detail here. You should, however, appreciate three things about contract damages. First, contract damages may not, and generally do not, equal the price of the contract. For example, if you renege on a deal to buy a new car for $35,000 from a car dealer, that dealer's damages under the law are most likely not $35,000. Second, damages in certain circumstances can be far greater than the contract price. For example, assume you reneged on a deal to sell 100 shares of stock to a friend for $5 per share. The stock then rises to $200 per share the day after the purchase and sale agreement for the stock is signed. In this case, you could be legally liable for far more than the $500 value of the contract for sale. Third, and perhaps most importantly, professional and general liability insurance usually does not insure you for breach of contract. If you are sued for breach, you will probably be personally liable.

Important Contractual Clauses

The key to contracts is the language that appears in them. Most contracts are broken down into numbered paragraphs or clauses. In an effort to assert some control over the outcome of disputes stemming from their contracts, parties include various clauses in their contracts. There are several of these clauses that typically appear in all types of formal written contracts. You need to have a basic understanding of the significance of such "boilerplate" clauses. These clauses containing "legalese" can have a significant impact upon the rights of the parties. They are discussed in the following subsections.

CHOICE OF FORUM CLAUSE

A *choice of forum* clause sets forth in advance the forum or court in which a lawsuit involving the contract may be brought. Because more than one court may have jurisdiction (power to hear a case), a forum selection clause prevents what is known as "forum shopping" by the parties' lawyers. An example of a choice of forum clause is as follows.

Box 16.1

Choice of Forum Clause
The parties agree that all disputes arising out of this contract shall be tried in the courts of New York State, to the exclusion of all other courts that might otherwise have jurisdiction apart from this contract provision.

A forum selection clause has several advantages. First, it limits the parties' exposure to courts in other jurisdictions, thereby saving costs and fees associated with travel to other states. Second, parties can avoid litigation in those states that are known for high jury awards.

Freely negotiated choice of forum clauses that are not designed to discourage litigation are generally upheld by courts. If a forum selection clause is rendered unenforceable, it does not mean that the contract itself is unenforceable. In such cases, the clause will simply be severed from the agreement, thereby allowing the plaintiff to bring a suit in any court that has jurisdiction. What you should remember is that by signing a contract that includes a choice of forum clause, you may be assenting to being sued in a distant state should a dispute arise. This could be very costly and inconvenient.

CHOICE OF LAW CLAUSE

Just because parties designate the location of the court that has power to resolve their dispute does not necessarily mean that the court will apply the law of the jurisdiction in which it is located. Thus, under certain circumstances, a Florida court may be required to apply New York law to decide a case. To prevent this from happening (or in some cases to ensure that this does happen) parties can insert a contractual clause that specifies the particular state's law that will govern their dispute. Such a clause is referred to as a *choice of law* clause.

Like a forum selection clause, choice of law clauses are generally enforceable if they are freely negotiated (i.e., not the result of fraud, duress, or undue influence). Another limitation is that the chosen state's law must be reasonably related to the transaction in order to be upheld. For example, the location of an office of one of the parties in the chosen state would be sufficient to uphold the clause. Box 16.2 contains an example of a choice of law clause found in a physician asset purchase agreement. Because the law of contracts varies from state to state, such clauses can have significant impact should a dispute arise.

Box 16.2

Choice of Law Clause
Buyer and Seller agree that this contract together with the rights and obligations of the parties shall be construed under and governed by the law of the state of Illinois.

ARBITRATION CLAUSE

Alternative forms of dispute resolution (ADR) are increasingly popular substitutes for formal civil litigation. *Arbitration*, the most common form of ADR, has the following advantages over litigation.

> 1. It's faster. It is not uncommon for a lawsuit to take years to come to trial.[1] The appeals process can add years to a final resolution of the dispute. The average time from filing date to a decision in an arbitrated dispute is 145 days.
> 2. It's cheaper. Lawyers charge by the hour, which becomes quite expensive if the litigation process drags on. Arbitration also avoids court costs, but does involve a private fee schedule.

---

[1] In 1988 there were approximately 17 million cases initiated in state and federal courts. See *State Court Caseload Statistics: Annual Report 3* (1989).

3. <u>It provides more control</u>. The parties can create a list from which the arbitrator is chosen. In litigation the judge is assigned. Also, the arbitrator is constrained by neither precedent nor the rules of evidence. He or she may therefore be able to tailor the result according to the facts presented. The parties can also agree on high-low or non-binding arbitration.

4. <u>It provides expert arbitrators</u>. The arbitrators are not required to be judges. They almost always have expertise in the field involving the dispute, and thus may be better suited to resolving complicated or technical issues than a judge who has been randomly assigned.

5. <u>It provides confidentiality</u>. The pleadings involved in a lawsuit are generally public record. Documents submitted with respect to an arbitrated dispute are not subject to public disclosure.

Arbitration decisions, also referred to as *awards*, are legally binding on parties who voluntarily submit to the process by including an arbitration clause in their contract. Courts may review arbitration awards, but such review is limited to procedural aspects such as fairness of the process and neutrality of the arbitrator. Courts generally will not undertake a review of the merits of the case. Box 16.3 is an example of an arbitration clause regarding the provision of medical treatment to a patient. What you need to be aware of is that by signing a contract that contains an arbitration clause, you are giving up your right to have future disputes under the contract litigated in a court of law before a jury.

Box 16.3

Arbitration Clause

It is understood that any dispute as to medical malpractice, that is as to whether any medical services rendered under this contract were unnecessary or unauthorized or were improperly, negligently or incompetently rendered, will be determined by submission to arbitration as provided by California law, and not by a lawsuit or resort to court except as California law provides for judicial review of arbitration proceedings. Both parties to this contract, by entering into it, are giving up their constitutional right to have any such dispute decided in a court of law before a jury, and instead are accepting the use of arbitration.[2]

INDEMNITY CLAUSES

To *indemnify* means to reimburse or restore a loss already incurred. In a contractual sense, an *indemnity* clause requires one party to reimburse the other for past or future losses. Such clauses are designed to shift the entire loss from one party who may be technically at fault to another who is primarily at fault. These clauses are commonly referred to as "hold harmless" clauses because one party is held responsible for damages or losses sustained as a result of the other party's fault. Depending upon the wording of an indemnity clause, such a clause could subject a person to substantial and uncontrollable risk, regardless of fault. You need to be very careful before signing a contract that calls on you to indemnify the other party. You should always seek, where possible, to have the other party agree to

---

[2] Language recommended by California Civil Code, section 1295.

indemnify you. An example of an indemnity clause follows.

Box 16.4

Indemnity Clause

Provider agrees to defend, indemnify and hold Managed Care Company harmless from and against any and all damages, liabilities, losses and expenses (including attorneys' fees) which in any way may arise from this agreement.

LIMITATION OF LIABILITY CLAUSE

A contract may contain a clause that states that one of the parties shall not be liable for breach. This type of clause is called a *limitation of liability* or an *exculpatory* clause. An exculpatory clause that attempts to excuse a party from liability in the case of intentional or reckless conduct is almost always unenforceable. Even clauses that purport to excuse ordinary negligence are not always binding. The purpose behind the court's unwillingness to enforce such clauses is that the law of torts has been created to protect others from the unreasonable risk of harm. Therefore, if such limitation of liability clauses were always enforceable, parties would be able to circumvent the standards of conduct imposed to protect the safety of others. The inclusion of an exculpatory clause in a contract by your opponent can be used against him if you argue that such a clause proves a lack of good faith.

COVENANTS NOT TO COMPETE

Covenants not to compete are frequently included in physician employment agreements.

Such agreements serve as a restraint of trade and will be closely scrutinized by the courts. To be enforceable, the clause must generally meet the following requirements.

> 1. It is reasonably necessary to protect a legitimate interest.
> 2. It does not impose an undue hardship to the promisor.
> 3. It is not likely to injure the public.

The term *reasonable* is hard to quantify because it depends upon the circumstances (such as size and nature of the business), but courts will examine the geographic scope and duration of the restraint in determining whether to enforce it. Box 16.5 contains a typical physician's covenant not to compete.

Box 16.5

Covenant Not to Compete

Neither he/she, nor any professional association, partnership, or practitioner of medicine with whom the Physician is currently or may in the future associate, will open, own, operate or otherwise participate in any emergency center, emergency clinic, general or family or any similar practice with in five (5) miles of any such emergency clinic or emergency center operated by EPS or any of its affiliates.

The Physician hereby agrees not to contract to provide services (or otherwise accept employment) with any facility which has had a contract with EPS, or any affiliate of EPS for a period of one (1) year following termination of such contract at the facility.

LIQUIDATED DAMAGES CLAUSES

As discussed above, the law of contract damages is extremely complicated. In some cases it may be difficult or even impossible to calculate the damages suffered by an injured party. Rather than leave this task to a jury, parties may insert a clause into their agreement that fixes the damages at a certain amount. This clause is known as a *liquidated damages* provision because it specifies in advance the amount of damages to be awarded in the case of breach. To be enforceable, the liquidated damages clause must generally provide for damages in an amount that is reasonable in light of the anticipated or actual loss caused by the breach. Additionally, the damages at the time of the loss need to be difficult to prove. A term fixing unreasonably large liquidated damages as a penalty is unenforceable on the grounds of public policy.

Notice that the amount must be *reasonable*. This is because the damages must not be punitive (penalizing) in nature, but instead must be designed to compensate the injured party. Consequently, excessive liquidated damages clauses will be unenforceable. Box 16.6 contains a liquidated damages clause.

Box 16.6

Liquidated Damages Clause
In the event of a material breach of the agreement, the party breaching the agreement shall be liable for $50,000 liquidated damages. This clause is intended as full and final liquidated damages for the material breach and the parties mutually agree that this amount does not constitute a penalty.

If the clause is enforceable, the effect of a liquidated damages clause is to allow the injured party to recover nothing more than the amount stipulated in the clause. Upon a showing of breach, the injured party is entitled to the specified amount regardless of whether the actual damages were more or less than the liquidated sum.

FORCE MAJEURE

A *force majeure* clause expresses the parties' intention that certain specified events, such as strikes and acts of God, shall excuse performance of the contract. Inclusion of such a clause helps alleviate the problems associated with relying on the doctrines of impossibility and impracticability. A sample force majeure clause follows.

Box 16.7

Force Majeure

Neither party shall be deemed to be in violation of this agreement if it is prevented from performing any of its obligations hereunder for any reason beyond its control, including, without limitation, strikes, inmate disturbances, acts of God, civil or military authority, acts of public enemy, or accidents, fires, explosions, earthquakes, floods, winds, failure of public transportation, or any other similar serious cause beyond the reasonable control of either party.

SEVERABILITY

A *severability* clause operates to preserve the remainder of a contract where one or more provisions, such as a choice of law or choice of forum clause, has been stricken by a court. The problem with such clauses is that the enforcement of the contract without the stricken clause or clauses may be problematic for the parties. A sample severability clause follows.

Box 16.8

Severability
If any provision contained in this agreement is held to be unenforceable by a court of law or equity, this agreement shall be construed as if such provision did not exist and the nonenforceability of such provision shall not be held to render any other provision or provisions of this agreement unenforceable.

NOTICE

Contracts frequently specify information or requests that need to be conveyed from one party to another. The form that such communication needs to take may be governed by a *notices* clause. An example of such a clause is provided in Box 16.9. When negotiating a contract, you need to make sure that you will be able to, and in fact do, comply with its notice provisions.

Box 16.9

Notices
All notices or other communications required or permitted to be given under this agreement shall be in writing and shall be deemed to have been duly given if delivered personally in hand, by telephonic facsimile or mailed certified mail, return receipt requested, postage prepaid on the date posted and addressed to the appropriate party.

ASSIGNMENT

An *assignment* involves one party transferring its rights and/or obligations under a contract to another party. Contracts frequently contain clauses governing each party's ability to do this. An example of such a clause follows.

Box 16.10

Assignment
Neither party shall assign, transfer, nor delegate any rights, obligations, or duties under this contract without the prior written consent of the other party.

TERMINATION

Most contracts contain a clause specifying how and when the contract is terminated. If you want to get out of a bad contractual relationship, this will be the crucial clause. An example of such a clause is provided in Box 16.11.

Box 16.11

Termination by Provider
Provider may terminate this agreement at any time, with or without cause, upon sixty (60) days prior written notice to Managed Care Company.

Non-form Contracts

Many important written contracts will not involve your being presented with standard form contracts. This may occur with employment contracts, medical practice purchase and sale contracts, and business contracts. When negotiating and drafting such contracts, you should involve an attorney. You need to keep in mind that you will be at a tremendous advantage if your attorney, as opposed to your opponent's attorney, prepares the first draft of the agreement. If she does, then the contract's fine print will be most favorable to you. Your opponent will then have to negotiate back from this draft. It could be very difficult for your opponent to subsequently negotiate away the fine print. The disadvantage to having your attorney draft the contract (subject to your opponent's review) is that you will typically incur greater legal costs. These costs stem from the increased time required to draft, as opposed to review, the first contract and the time required to make any and all changes to future drafts.

When your attorney does not or cannot draft the original contract, you will often receive a one-sided document favorable to your opponent. There are ways to defend against this. First, you can respond that you are taken aback by such a one-sided document and threaten to use your alternatives. Second, you can use the promise of a long-term relationship to seek to make the contract fairer. Third, you can simply state that you do not sign complicated contracts and demand that your opponent come back with a simpler document. Finally, remember that when negotiating any contractual term you always need to have a credible rationale for why it should be included or excluded. You should also look carefully for potential ambiguities and always ask yourself "what if." The time to resolve "what if" questions is when the contract is being negotiated, not when something goes wrong at a later date. Consider the following examples.

Example 16.1

Doctor: I thought you were acting in good faith until I saw that contract that your lawyer sent over. You expect me to indemnify you for your *own* negligence and disclaim liability for any and all harm caused. And what's this about $50,000 in liquidated damages? I never agreed to any of that. I'm negotiating with three other doctors for shared use of my office space. None of them would ever come up with a document like this.

Opponent: I'm sorry, I didn't know. I'll have to have a talk with my lawyer. Why don't you have your lawyer make whatever changes you feel are necessary and send it over directly to me?

Lesson: Through the controlled use of emotion (see pages 161-168 on emotion) and a good rationale ("I never agreed to that"), the doctor was able to do a good job in negotiating changes to the terms of the contract. The implied threat of dealing with someone else was also helpful.

Example 16.2

Doctor: I'm looking for a long-term relationship here. Our practice is expanding, and we'd love to stay in this property if we are treated fairly. We may even need to take over more floors in the very near future. This clause requiring written permission to make any and all alterations to the leased premises isn't going to work. And the $40,000 liquidated damages provision is patently unfair. What would happen if you rented the same space the next day for a higher rent? This lease is about the future and should be a basis of our future agreements. We need a fair document that protects both sides. This isn't it.

Opponent: I'm in it for the long term too and would love to have you. Let's make it work for both of us. Strike out those clauses and fax it back to me.

Lesson: The rationale of fairness and reasonableness can be effective when demanding changes to a written contract. Furthermore, it is *always* to your benefit to communicate that you will be seeking to negotiate with your opponent again in the future.

Example 16.3

Doctor: I received your 17-page contract and, to be honest, I was a little taken aback. This isn't a complicated deal and it shouldn't take 17 pages to cover it. I'm not paying a lawyer thousands of dollars to review it. Send over something that's one or two pages long and then we'll talk.

Opponent: My lawyer says that we need this 17-pager to protect us.

Doctor: Are you saying you don't trust me? If you and your lawyer really think that you need a 17-page, one-sided document to protect yourself from me, then we probably shouldn't be doing business at all.

Opponent: I didn't mean to imply that at all. Let me draft something much simpler, have my lawyer review it, then send it over to you.

Lesson: If your opponent's lawyer is drafting the contract, it is usually in your best interest to have the contract be as short as possible. This is true because most, if not all, of the additional language will be in the contract for your opponent's benefit and your detriment.

Example 16.4

Doctor: The contract you sent over states that I will be responsible to take call "on a rotating basis." That is ambiguous. This could mean that I take call every other night and weekend. Let's add a sentence that states, "In no event shall employee be required to take call more than one night per week and one weekend per month."

Opponent: Fine. Mark up the document in red and I'll have my lawyer run the change.

Lesson: The doctor had a good rationale for correcting the possible ambiguity. It would be difficult for his opponent to refuse to allow the addition of the requested language because he would be less likely to come up with a rationale while still appearing to negotiate in good faith.

Example 16.5

Doctor: One final thing. Let's add a force majeure clause that says that if I die or become disabled before the closing date, I, or my estate, will be excused from purchasing your practice.

Opponent: Well, let's hope that doesn't happen. Sure.

Lesson: The time to protect yourself from a possible bad turn of events is before the contract is signed. You have the power to plan for and protect yourself from certain contingencies. Think hard about your contracts and use that power.

Example 16.6

Doctor: We need to talk about this covenant not to compete. I agree that you need to protect yourself.

However, you stated during my interview that over 90% of your patients are within a five-mile radius of your clinic. The covenant in this contract restricts me to areas outside of 20 miles from the practice. That's unfair, overbroad, and unnecessary to give you proper protection.

Opponent: Okay. We'll make it five miles.

Lesson: During the interview the doctor gained valuable information, which she then used during negotiations over the formal written contract. (See pages 39-82 and 122-126 on information.) The doctor was savvy enough to realize that that initial interview was part of the negotiation process. By conceding that the clinic needs protection, the doctor helped strengthen her rationale that the clause was overbroad and unnecessary. The doctor did not rely on the courts to conclude on some later date that the clause was overbroad. She successfully negotiated away potentially costly future problems.

Negotiating Standard Form Contracts

Many contracts today are standard form contracts. Standard form contracts include leases, managed care contracts, and consumer contracts, for example for the purchase and sale of an automobile. Applicable state law may give relief from some form contracts if something goes wrong. You *cannot* rely on obtaining such relief. You should try to negotiate more favorable terms even in standard form contracts. It can be done!

You will never get a change made to a standard form contract unless you ask for it. Due to the power of legitimacy (see pages 110-112 on legitimacy), many physicians do not even attempt to negotiate standard or form contracts. When you do ask for changes, you will need to have a rationale that is strong enough to justify the changes. Your opponents may indeed have the authority to amend their form contracts. The same rules apply for non-form contracts. You will need to review the contracts carefully for ambiguities and carefully consider "what if" problems. You also can use the possibility of a long-term relationship and your other alternatives to gain power in the negotiation and changes in the standard contract. Don't be afraid to give the impression that you are prepared to walk away. This impression may work to make your opponent a lot more flexible. Consider the following examples.

Example 16.7
Doctor: Your company gets access under clause 6.2 to my patients' medical records. I will need you to add a clause stating that the plan will reimburse me for my expenses in copying these records.
Opponent: That's not part of the standard contract.
Doctor: That's not my concern. What's to stop you from frequently requesting voluminous medical records when you don't know exactly what you are looking for? Why should I have to pick up the cost if you do? Under managed care I am supposed to accept incentives to become more efficient, so why shouldn't you?
Opponent: What language do you propose...?

Lesson: The doctor was not afraid to ask for a change in the standard contract after his "what if" analysis detected a potential problem with medical record requests. He was prepared with a powerful rationale to justify the requested change.

Example 16.8
Doctor: This provider agreement can only be terminated on 180 days advance notice. That's far too long. The other providers I am negotiating with all call for 60-day termination periods. That's the industry standard. You're looking for a long-term provider in this area and I want a long-term relationship with a provider who is in line with accepted practices.
Opponent: Cross out the 180 and insert 60.

Lesson: The doctor was not afraid to ask for a change. She used her alternatives (other managed care companies) and the possibility of a long-term relationship to gain power in the negotiation. The industry standard was a powerful rationale for her requested change. Note that her opponent did indeed have the authority to change the language in the standard contract.

Example 16.9
Opponent: Doctor, we haven't heard from you in two weeks. I just wanted to follow up on the status of negotiations.
Doctor: (sounding cold and noncommittal) Well, as you recall, I had some serious concerns about that standard agreement you sent over.
Opponent: (after a moment of silence) Ahh..., that's why I'm calling. I want to work with you so that we can get an agreement that's fair to both of us.
Doctor: Okay then. First, remove....

Lesson: Your opponent may be bluffing when she gives you the impression that she has no flexibility in negotiating the contract. She may very well have flexibility. Furthermore, even when you think you need the deal more than your opponent, this may not be the case. A failure to get back to your opponent in a timely manner may communicate that you do not need the deal and may help you gain power in the negotiation.

Chapter 17 Closing the Deal

The final step in any negotiation is closing the deal. There are a series of closing techniques that can be used to help close a deal. These include the assumptive close, linkage, the clear choice, and the power of investment. You need to understand when you have a deal and the importance of "face saving" to your opponent. Finally, when closing the deal you will want to ensure that an ongoing or potential long-term relationship is not jeopardized and is in fact strengthened by the closing.

Assumptive Close

The successful physician negotiator recognizes when he or she has "won over" the opponent and an agreement is at hand. When the agreement is very close to being reached, the assumptive close is an appropriate technique to finalize the deal. The *assumptive close* involves your "assuming" that a deal has been reached and concluded. This psychological closing tactic forces your opponent to either say, "No, you are wrong. We have no deal" (which, at the very end of a negotiation, is difficult to do), or to accept the fact that the agreement has been reached. Calling third parties, for example, lawyers, accountants, or spouses, is another affirmation that the agreement has in fact been finalized. This closing tactic is very effective when all the major terms have been worked out but the opponent is having difficulty concluding the negotiation and saying the words, "We have a deal."

Example 17.1
Doctor: (to opponent) Excellent! All of our hard work has paid off! I will call the venture capital people and tell them to start the paperwork. You can use my office, line three, to call your parties.

Lesson: The doctor has forced his opponent's hand. The opponent now needs to either assent to the deal or explain to the doctor why he is not assenting.

Linkage

One of the most effective methods of increasing the psychological pressure to achieve an agreement is linkage. (See pages 142-144 on linkage.) Linkage in this context involves a quid pro quo in the form of a concession in exchange for finalizing the agreement.

Example 17.2
Hospital recruiter: (to prospective doctor employee) Doctor, as you know, we would welcome you to the faculty. The only remaining issue is the salary.
Doctor: It usually is.
Hospital recruiter: As I have mentioned repeatedly, our salary structure is such that we cannot exceed a starting salary of $140,000. Keep in mind that we have already agreed to your four weeks of vacation, health, disability, and malpractice insurance, cell phone, pager, and relocation expenses.
Doctor: We appreciate all the perks, but I need $150,000.
Hospital recruiter: Our salary structure is such....
Doctor: If I agreed to sign a letter of intent today, would you put in a $10,000 signing bonus? This would

maintain your salary structure and give me and my family what we need.

Hospital recruiter: Let me make one quick call…. We have a deal!

Lesson: The doctor has listened carefully to the final objection (see pages 64-82 on active listening) and has overcome the objection by linkage. His willingness to consent to finalize the deal was a concession that gained him $10,000.

Clear Choice

The clear choice closing tactic can also be useful in finalizing an agreement. The clear choice tactic involves focusing your opponent's choices in such a way that closing the deal is the best option available to her. When you know you may be losing some time or money, the "clear choice" option can help cut your losses.

Example 17.3

Salesperson: The options are leasing the copying equipment for two years at $600 a month, or leasing it for three years at $500 a month and locking in the price for the additional year, or purchasing the equipment outright for $15,000.

Doctor: Why should I lease for two or three years when I could just purchase the equipment outright for the same price? At least this way I own the equipment.

Salesperson: Not many people have your grasp of finances, doctor. Let me write up the sales agreement. For signing today, I will throw in one year of service and all the copy paper I have in my Geo. Just don't tell all the other doctors in this medical complex the deal that you got!

Lesson: The salesperson effectively focused the doctor's choices and then made the decision easy and inevitable.

Example 17.4
Doctor: (to staff members) You have the option of taking off the day before Christmas, New Year's, Thanksgiving, or July 4th, which comes on a Saturday. Please pass around a sign-up sheet. As you know, we cannot close down on those days due to our patients and the $5,000 a day we have in overhead.

Lesson: By limiting her opponent's choices, the doctor has made the closing of a deal more likely.

Power of Investment

The power of investment (see pages 108-109 on investment) can also be used as an effective closing technique. When you point out your opponent's investment in a negotiation, it makes it much more difficult for him to walk away from the deal.

Example 17.5
Physician head of nonprofit organization: (to prospective doctor author) Your idea for a book is viable...however, due to the fact that we are a nonprofit association and have our own publications, I am not sure if we can proceed.

Doctor: (appearing overeager) Well, I know the book will be excellent. As you know, I am the leading authority on the subject.

Physician: Doctor, your credentials are impeccable. No one here questions even for a moment your abilities. If we did, we would not have let you prepare the twenty-page outline, spend $847 in airfare, $180 in hotel expenses, and lose two days of work to come here to discuss the project.

Doctor: As you know, I have been working on this concept, outline, and even a few chapters....

Physician: I don't want to see you come away empty handed after all the time, money, and effort you have spent. We can authorize "our" book. We will retain the copyright, set the price, be solely in charge of the marketing and the supplements, and we will give you a 10% royalty payable twelve months after the end of our fiscal year, which is June 15th. We want the book as soon as possible.

Doctor: Thank you. I will get right on it.

Lesson: The doctor revealed to her opponent her investment in the negotiation. By doing so she revealed damaging information. Her opponent used this investment against her to close an unfavorable deal.

Having a Deal

Making a deal or having a deal means having an agreement on all outstanding issues, obtaining a written memorandum of agreement without ambiguities, and reaching an agreement that can and will be lived up to by all parties.

OUTSTANDING ISSUES

After a lengthy and/or a complex negotiation session, it is common for the parties to later run into problems when some of the terms have not been spelled out in detail. You should not consider a deal closed until all details have been worked out. This means that you should not take steps that could be detrimental to you if the deal falls through until all outstanding issues have been finalized. Prematurely considering a deal closed can be very dangerous.

Example 17.6
Proposed employer: (to new doctor employee) We are all set. I will tell our attorneys to draw up the employment contract and you can have your attorney review it.
Doctor: Great! I look forward to starting on Monday.
Employer: Actually, you start this Saturday. Under our call coverage plan, you work this weekend. You get every other weekend off and you cover at the emergency department every seventh day. Also, you have to cover the clinic at night.
Doctor: Wait just a minute. You never mentioned and I never agreed to this....
Employer: Actually, if you remember, we agreed that you would have the same call coverage as the other physicians.... This is what everyone is doing. You are a team player, aren't you doctor?
Doctor: Yes...but...I already told my spouse we had an agreement. I have to call her right away. She was going to give her two weeks notice today at work.

Lesson: This doctor acted on the deal before all outstanding issues were finalized. He might now be stuck with a deal he would have otherwise walked away from.

WRITTEN MEMORANDA AND CONTRACTS

When it comes time to write up a memorandum of agreement, contract, or letter of intent, the party who took detailed and clear notes during the negotiation is in the position of power. Also remember that the party whose attorney drafts the initial agreement will also be in a position of power. This is because the fine print in the initial draft will favor the client of the attorney who drafted the agreement. The opponent's counsel will then be in a position of negotiating back from that agreement. The downside to having your attorney draft the contract is that when this is done, you will generally incur greater legal expenses than your opponent.

Example 17.7
Doctor: Just to summarize, you are looking for $1,000 a month retainer. For the $1,000 you will draft and copy both print and radio ads, place the copy, and determine the cost-efficiency of the ads.
Marketing group leader: That is correct.
Doctor: There are no additional or hidden charges to us.
Marketing group leader: That's right... one flat fee.
Doctor: Your group will not be paid anything over and above the $1,000 a month, right?
Marketing group leader: Well, it will not cost you anything else, but we do get the standard 20% ad agency commission.
Doctor: That should come back to us. We agreed to $1,000 a month....
Marketing group leader: It is standard practice for all agencies to retain the 20%.

Doctor: My notes of the negotiation session are clear. Your group gets $1,000 a month, no additional fees. If you will not live up to the agreement you just made, we really can't do business with your group.

Marketing group leader: To be fair to us, this commission issue was not clearly spelled out by either party. We assumed we would retain it and you assumed, apparently, that if there was any commission that it would revert to you.

Doctor: We need to straighten out this ambiguity and any other ones before we can sign the contract.

Lesson: Accurate notes helped the doctor gain power in the negotiation.

LIVING UP TO THE AGREEMENT

Any agreement or contract is only as good as the people who sign it. A party's intention and ability to live up to the agreement is critical. If you can demonstrate a track record of living up to agreements you have made in the past, you will be more likely to close the deal.

Example 17.8

Medical education company representative: You are our choice to help produce a video on informed consent, doctor.

Doctor: As I mentioned, I am very interested in the project.

Medical education company representative: We have set up a time line of three months to produce a final script and three months to shoot and edit the video. We are looking for twenty minutes.

Doctor: As you know, I have written thirty-six papers on informed consent and have lectured internationally on the subject. I was thinking I could have a final script done in two weeks and have the whole project wrapped up in one month. The video should be sixty minutes long.

Medical education company representative: We want to have realistic time frames, doctor. We have produced fourteen videos like this. Our experience has been that it takes two or three times as long as you would think. We have to line up a producer and director, and reserve sets and equipment. We need to be sure that we give you enough time so you can produce the work without falling behind schedule. Every hour we spend in pre-production saves us three hours in filming. We need only twenty high quality minutes.

Doctor: I will trust your judgment. You have the experience. Let's go with the six-month timeline and twenty-minute video.

Lesson: The company was able to use its track record to gain a concession from the doctor and close a deal.

Face Saving

If there is any chance that you may be dealing with your opponent again in the future, it is important for her to come out of the negotiating session looking good to her superior or employer. (See pages 147-148 on "the story.") You should use the close of a deal as an opportunity to make your opponent look good. If you do, your future negotiations are more likely to be resolved favorably. As a corollary to this principle, you should never gloat or be demeaning at the end of a negotiation. Doing so serves no purpose and can be very detrimental to future negotiations and dealings.

Example 17.9
Doctor: (on the phone to the negotiator's superior after a tough negotiation) I just want to congratulate you on your employee, Ms. Bonds. In the twenty-five years I have been a physician, she was the most effective negotiator I ever faced. She listened, dealt with my concerns and issues, and was tough but fair. I don't think anyone else could have gotten me to sign the contract on those terms. Even after so nicely beating my terms into the ground, she was so pleasant that I couldn't even be upset at all. I gave up. I look forward to doing business with you and my worthy adversary, Ms. Bonds, in the future.

Lesson: Ms. Bonds will hear about the kind comments and will be more likely to go out of her way to make sure future negotiations go smoothly.

Example 17.10
Doctor: (to opponent by fax after negotiation) It was good doing business with you. Just as a point of information, I would have taken 30% less and still signed the contract.

Lesson: There is *no* efficacy to this fax. The doctor has made it much more difficult for himself if he ever needs to negotiate in the future.

An Alternative Approach

One way to encourage your opponent to finalize a deal is to stress your alternatives should a deal not be reached. Your opponent may often try to delay or think over a deal for as long as possible out of a hope to gain further concessions. By employing the technique of stressing alternatives, you can motivate your opponent to close the deal. She will be motivated to do so if further delay can be objectively demonstrated as being likely to make you deal with another party, thus leaving your opponent without any deal.

Example 17.11
Orthopedic surgeon: (to prospective physician employee) We have been negotiating for three weeks. I have listened very carefully to all your needs and have gone beyond my authority to try and meet almost each and every one of them. My partners have instructed me to reach an agreement today by 5:00 P.M. or else re-open our search efforts in order to recruit another orthopedic surgeon. If we can't reach a memorandum of understanding today, we will start the second interviews of other qualified and interested candidates.

Lesson: By stressing her alternatives, the doctor has gained power in the negotiation and made a timely closing of the deal more likely.

Example 17.12
Doctor: We enjoyed the few days you have spent with us. The negotiation has been challenging but educational. We have put our best offer on the table. Sometimes when you are just starting out, it is hard to tell when someone is bending over backwards to be fair. Why don't you take all the time you need to think it over? In the meantime, we will invite several other doctors who are very interested in this opportunity to work in our office.
Prospective hire: May I call my wife? I do not need any additional time to think it over.

Lesson: By using a bit of reverse psychology and stressing the practice's alternatives, the doctor was able to push his opponent into making a decision.

Resources

Author(s):	Churchman, David
Title:	*Negotiation Tactics*
Edition & date:	1993
ISBN:	0-819-19164-7 (alk. paper)/ 0-819-1916-55 (paper: alk. paper)
Publisher:	Lanham, MD: University Press of America
Price:	$29.50

Author(s):	Cohen, Herb
Title:	*You Can Negotiate Anything*
Edition & date:	1st ed./1980
ISBN:	0-8184-0305-5
Publisher:	Secaucus, NJ: L. Stuart
Price:	$12.00

Author(s):	Cohen, Herb
Title:	*You Can Negotiate Anything*
Edition & date:	1995
ISBN:	0-8065-0847-7
Publisher:	Secaucus, N.J.: Carol Publishing Group
Price:	$10.95

Author(s):	Craver, Charles B.
Title:	*Effective Legal Negotiation and Settlement*
Edition & date:	2nd ed./1993
ISBN:	1-55834-059-9

Publisher: Massachusetts Continuing Legal
                   Education, Inc.
Price: $65.00

Author(s):   DK Publishing, Inc.
Title: *Negotiate Successfully*
Edition & date: 1st American ed./1998
ISBN: 0-7894-2448-7
Publisher: New York: DK Pub.
Price: Contact supplier for piece
                   information

Author(s):   Donaldson, Michael C./
                   Mimi Donaldson
Title: *Negotiating for Dummies*
Edition & date: 1st ed./1996
ISBN: 1-56884-867-6
Publisher: Chicago: IDG Books Worldwide
Price: $19.99 (USA)/$26.99 (Canada)

Author(s):   Fisher, Roger/Ertel, Danny
Title: *Getting Reading to Negotiate*
Edition & date: 1995
ISBN: 0-14-023531-0
Publisher: New York: Penguin Books
Price: $12.95 (USA)/$16.99 (Canada)

Author(s):   Fisher, Roger
Title: *Getting Ready to Negotiate:*
                   The Getting to Yes Workbook
Edition & date: 1995
ISBN: 0-14-023531-0

Publisher: New York: Penguin Books
Price:

Author(s):   Fisher, Roger/William Ury
                   (Bruce Patton, ed.)
Title: *Getting to Yes: Negotiating*
                   Agreement Without Giving In
Edition & date: Rev. ed./1991
ISBN: 0-395-31757-6
Publisher: Boston: Houghton Mifflin
Price: $12.95

Author(s):   Fisher, Roger/William Ury
                   (Bruce Patton, ed.)
Title: *Getting to Yes: Negotiating*
                   Agreement Without Giving In
Edition & date: 2nd ed./1991
ISBN: 0-14-015735-2
Publisher: New York: Penguin Books
Price: $8.95

Author(s):   Fleming, Peter
Title: *Successful Negotiating*
Edition & date: 1st ed./1997
ISBN: 0-7641-0125-0
Publisher: New York: Barron's Educational
                   Series, Inc.
Price: $6.95 (USA)/$8.95 (Canada)

Author(s):   Gresser, Julian
Title: *Piloting through Chaos:*

	Wise Leadership, Effective Negotiation for the 21st Century
Edition & date:	1st ed./1996
ISBN:	1888278005 (alk. paper)
Publisher:	Sausalito, CA: Five Rings Press
Price:	$19.95 (paper)

Author(s):	Hall, Lavinia
Title:	*Negotiation: Strategies for Mutual Gain: The Basic Seminar of the Harvard Program on Negotiation*
Edition & date:	1992
ISBN:	0-8039-4849-2 (hard)/ 0-8039-4850-6 (paper)
Publisher:	Newbury Park, CA: SagePublications
Price:	$48.00

Author(s):	Ilich, John
Title:	*The Complete Idiot's Guide to: Winning through Negotiation*
Edition & date:	1996
ISBN:	0-02-861037-7
Publisher:	New York: Alpha Books
Price:	$16.95 (USA)/$23.95 (Canada)

Author(s):	Jandt, Fred E.
Title:	*Win-Win Negotiating*
Edition & date:	1st ed./1985
ISBN:	0-471-85877-3 (paper)
Publisher:	New York: John Wiley & Sons
Price:	$19.95

Author(s):   Johnson, Ralph A.
Title: *Negotiation Basics: Concepts, Skills, and Exercises*
Edition & date: 1993
ISBN: 0-8039-4051-3 (cloth)/
                        0-8039-4052-1 (paper)
Publisher: CA: Newbury Park
                        Sage Publications
Price: $16.95 (paper)

Author(s):   Karrass, Chester Louis
Title: *Give and Take: The Complete Guide to Negotiating Strategies and Tactics*
Edition & date: Rev. ed./1993
ISBN: 0-88730-606-3
Publisher: New York: Harper Business
Price: $25.00 (cloth)/$33.50 (Canada)

Author(s):   Karrass, Chester Louis
Title: *In Business As in Life—You Don't Get What You Deserve, You Get What You Negotiate*
Edition & date: 1st ed./1996
ISBN: 0-9652274-9-9
Publisher: Los Angeles: Stanford
                        Street Press
Price: $29.50

Author(s):   Karrass, Chester Louis
Title: *The Negotiating Game*
Edition & date: Rev. ed./1994
ISBN: 0-88730-568-7

Publisher: New York: HarperCollins
Price: $20.00 (USA)/$26.75 (Canada)

Author(s):   Kennedy, Gavin
Title: *The Perfect Negotiation*
Edition & date: 1994
ISBN: 0517101432
Publisher: New York: Random House
                  Value
Price: $5.99

Author(s):   Lewicki, Roy J.
Title: *Essentials of Negotiation*
Edition & date: 1996
ISBN: 0-256-24168-6
Publisher: Chicago: Irwin
Price: $29.95

Author(s):   Lewicki, Roy J.
Title: *Negotiation: Reading, Exercises,
                  and Cases*
Edition & date: 3rd ed./1997
ISBN: 025621591X
Publisher: Boston: Irwin/McGraw-Hill
Price: $29.80

Author(s):   McCormack, Mark H.
Title: *What They Don't Teach You at
                  Harvard Business School: Notes
                  from a Street-Smart Executive*
Edition & date: 1986

ISBN: 0-553-34583-4
Publisher: New York: Bantam Books
Price: $14.95 (USA)/$19.95 (Canada)

Author(s):   McCormack, Mark H.
Title: *What They Still Don't Teach You
                   at Harvard Business School:
                   Selling More, Managing Better,
                   and Getting the Job Done in the
                   90s*
Edition & date: 1989
ISBN: 0-553-34961-9
Publisher: New York: Bantam Books
Price: $14.95 (USA)/$20.95 (Canada)

Author(s):   McMillan, John
Title: *Games, Strategies, & Managers*
Edition & date: 1st ed./1996
ISBN: 0-19-510803-5
Publisher: New York: Oxford University
                   Press
Price: $16.95

Author(s):   McRae, Brad
Title: *Negotiating & Influencing Skills:
                   The Art of Creating & Claiming
                   Value*
Edition & date: 1997
ISBN: 0-7619-1184-7
Publisher: Thousand Oaks, CA:
                   Sage Publications
Price:

Author(s):   Poulopoulos, Peter J.
Title: *Negotiating Tips: A Practical
                 Guide to Be a Successful
                 Negotiator and Obtain Results*
Edition & date: 1st ed./1996
ISBN:
Publisher: Chicago: Tanesoic Learning
                 Systems (2731 W. Touhy Ave.,
                 Chicago, 60645)
Price:

Author: Quinley, Kevin M.
Title: *Litigation Management*
Edition & date: 1st ed./1995
ISBN: 1-886813-00-0
Publisher: Dallas: International Risk
                 Management Institute, Inc.
Price:

Author(s):   Schaffzin, Nicholas Reid
Title: *Don't Be a Chump!*
Edition & date: 1st ed./1995
ISBN: 0-679-76130-6
Publisher: New York: Random House
                 Value
Price: $12.00

Author(s):   Schaffzin, Nicholas Reid
Title: *Negotiate Smart*
Edition & date: 1997
ISBN: 0-679-77871-3

Publisher: Princeton Review
                  Publishing, LLC; Random
Price: $12.00 (USA)/$16.95 (Canada)

Author(s):   Stark, Mike R.
Title: *The Power of Negotiating:*
                  Strategies for Success
Edition & date: 1996
ISBN: 0964945304
Publisher: Littleton, CO:
                  Trimark Publishing
Price: $12.95

Author(s):   Walker, Michael A.
Title: *Negotiations: Six Steps*
                  to Success
Edition & date: 1995
ISBN: 0131255924
Publisher: Upper Saddle River, NJ:
                  PTR Prentice Hall
Price: $19.95

Index

Accelerated deadlines, 92, 95, 101-102
Acceptance time, 83, 90-92
Active listening, 64-82, 127, 173-174, 207-208, 259
Agendas, 214-215
Alternatives, 105-106, 111, 116, 266-268
Ambush negotiations, 27-31, 85-87, 117-118, 183
Analysis, 126-129
Anchoring, 191-193
Answering questions, 57-64
Arbitration clause, 239-241
Asking questions, 48-57
Assertiveness, 13-17
Assignment clause, 247
Assumptions about opponents, flawed, 126-129
Assumptive close, 257-258
Attorney, retaining an, 217-234
Attorneys' fees, 220-228
    blended, 221
    contingency, 221-224
    fixed, 221, 224-225
    hourly, 221, 225-228
Auditory feedback, 169, 173-174, 175
Authority, 39-48, 146, 196, 210, 253
Avoiding deadlock, 150-160
Awards, 238, 240

Ballpark figure, 183-186, 226
Bargaining against yourself, 42, 43, 193-194
Belly up, 190-191
Bids, 198
Blended fees, 219, 220, 221
Body language, 48, 62, 71-74, 173
Break, during negotiations, 161, 205-207
Breaking deadlock, 149-160
Brinksmanship, 93, 198
Brooklyn approach, 51-52

Candor, lack of, 186-188
Caucusing, 205, 207, 208-210
Change, 156-160

Choice of forum clause, 237-238
Choice of law clause, 238-239
Clauses, contractual, 237-247
Clear choice, 259-260
Client, being a good, 231-233
Close deadlines, 97-98
Closing the deal, 42, 257-268
Competitive negotiation, 12, 13, 22-23, 159, 233
Composing a team, 201-202
Concentration, 169-170
Concessions, 11, 13, 41, 42, 43, 44, 77, 90, 92, 139-148, 177-179
 rate and size of, 145-147
 recognizing, 139-141
 the story of, 147-148, 265-266
 value of, 141-142
Conciliatory language, 150-151
Confirmation letter, 169, 174-175
Contingency fee, 221-224
Contract law, 235-237
Contracts,
 non-form, 247-252
 standard form, 252-255
Contractual clauses, 237-247
Contractual damages, 236-237
Controlled emotions, 127, 161-168, 249
Controlling the information flow, 202-204
Cooperative negotiation, 12-22, 23, 159, 233
Counsel selection, 233-234
Covenant not to compete clause, 242-243

Damages, contractual, 236-237
Deadlines, 92-102, 153-154
 accelerated, 92, 95, 101-102
 close, 97-98
 extension of, 99-101
 objective, 98-99
 power of, 94-95
Deadlock, 149-160
 breaking or avoiding, 150-160
 eliminating the possibility of, 154-155
Decision tree, 129-132
Decisions, deflecting, 28-29, 35-36
Declining questions, 58, 60

Deferring questions, 58, 60
Deflecting decisions, 28-29, 35-36
Deflecting questions, 58, 60
Delay, 42-43
Delaying questions, 58, 60
Desires of opponent, 74-82
Diagnosis of tactics, 177-189
Diffusing an opponent, 162-163
Disclosure of information, 34-35, 57-58
Divide and conquer, 211-212

Emotions, 127, 161-168, 249
Equivocal statements, 70
Estimates, 183-186, 226
Exculpatory clause, 242
Excuses not to negotiate, 7-9
Expenses, legal, 229-230
Expertise, 107-108
Extension of deadlines, 99-101

Face saving, 265-266
False flattery, 197
Fear, playing on, 95-96, 165-168, 193-194
Fees, legal, 220-228
Fixed legal fees, 221, 224-225
Flexibility, 112-113, 151-152, 205, 215
Flight back gambit, 84
Focus, 36-37, 169-170
Force majeure clause, 245
Formal written contracts, 235-255

Goals, 90-91, 120-122, 204-205
Goodwill, building, 20-21

Having a deal, 261-265
Hiring an attorney, 230-231
Home field advantage, 33-34
Home field disadvantage, 34-37
Hourly legal fees, 221, 225-228

Indemnity clauses, 241-242
Industry standards, 106-107
Information gathering, 39-82, 103-105, 122-126, 202-203, 251-252

Information, disclosure of, 34-35, 202-203
Initiating the call, 171-173
Interests of opponents, 74-82
Interruptions, 34
Investment, 108-109, 145, 146, 157, 260-261
Issues, identifying and defining, 119-120

Knowledge is power, 103-105

Lack of candor, 186-188
Law office economics, 217-220
Leading questions, 52-53
Legal fee arrangements, 220-228
Legitimacy, 110-112, 252-255
Letting people off the hook, 21-22
Limitation of liability clause, 242
Limited time offer, 198
Linkage, 142-144, 258-259
Liquidated damages clause, 244-245
Listening, active, 64-82, 127, 173-174
Living up to the agreement, 264-265
Location, 33-37, 129
Logistics, 36
Long-term relationships, benefits of, 19

Managed care contracts, 235, 252, 253, 254, 255
Maslow, Abraham, 75
Memoranda and contracts, 174, 261, 263-264

Needs of opponents, 18-19, 74-82, 103
Negotiation
    ambush, 27-31, 85-87, 117-118, 183
    competitive, 12, 13, 22-23, 159, 233
    cooperative, 12-22, 23, 159, 233
    defined, 11-12
    magic formula, 24
    principles, 24-25
Negotiations, team, 201-215
Non-form contracts, 247-252
Nonverbal communication, 48, 62, 71-74, 173, 207-208
Note taking, 169, 174-175, 207-208, 263
Notice clause, 246

Objective deadlines, 98-99
Outrageous opening offer, 189-190
Outstanding issues, 262-263

Patience, 87-88
Pausing, 88-90
Persistence, 113-114
Personalizing the negotiation, 164-165
Planning, 57, 117, 129-132
Playing dumb, 49-51
Playing it cool, 161-163
Pleading poverty, 194-195
Power, 11, 103-116
Power of investment, 260-261
Precedents, 110-112
Preparation, 36-37, 57, 103-105, 117-132, 170-171

Questions
    answering, 57-64
    asking, 48-57
    declining, 58, 60
    deferring, 58, 60
    delaying, 58, 60
    leading, 52-53
    successive, 52, 53-54
    suggestive, 52, 53
    what if, 52, 54-55
Quickie negotiations, 170

Recognizing concessions, 139-141
Reframing techniques, 67-68
Renegotiation, 199
Resolving team disagreements, 210-211
Reverse contingency fee, 221
Room to negotiate, 139, 152-153, 178-179

Saving face, 265-266
Saying no, 28-31
Selection from a limited menu, 199
Severability clause, 245-246
Signaling, 205-207
Silence, 133-137
Sole source, 115-116

Splitting the difference, 146, 177-179, 225
Stalling, 197
Standard form contracts, 252-255
Story of concessions, 147-148, 265-266
Successive questions, 52, 53-54
Suggestive questions, 52, 53

Tactics
    diagnosis and treatment of, 129, 177-199
    team negotiation, 211-214
Take it or leave it, 179-183
Tapping into fear or anxiety, 95-96, 165-168
Team disagreements, resolving, 210-211
Team negotiations, 201-215
Telephone negotiations, 169-175
Tempo, 136-137
Termination clause, 247
Timing, 83-102, 144-145
Treatment of tactics, 177-189
Trial balloon, 54, 140, 197
Trickle-down loss, 42, 44, 47
Trust, building, 17-18, 22

Ultimatums, 153-154
Uncertainty, 112-113

Verbal leaks, 65, 70, 135

Weak link, 212-214
Wedge, 211-212
What, 124-125
What if questions, 52, 54-55
What is *not* being said, 68-69, 127
When, 122-123
When to negotiate, 83-87
Where, 125
Who, 123-124
Why, 126
Why physicians don't negotiate, 7-9, 117
Win-win solution, 12, 16, 17, 19, 159, 174
Written proposals, 29-30

X factor, 77-82